CHARGE UP

How your body works
Why you feel the way you do
What you can do about it

Drs. Sherri and Stockton Jacobs ND, CNS
Creators of Clean UP and Tighten UP
Founders of HealthE Coaching

Resources and handouts for Charge UP can be found at: http://healthecoaching.com/charge-up-program/charge-up-additional-resources/

This book is dedicated with deep gratitude to our clients. It was through their great resolve, their pioneering spirit and their willingness to trust in our education and training that we developed the approach contained within this book. Thank you.

And, we dedicate this book to ourselves. Creating new ideas and taking risks for what you believe can be a lonely road. As a couple, and like so many of our clients, we have confronted many challenges in life, but we have come through stronger and closer. As a husband-wife team we remain deeply in love, best friends and lucky parents. As clinicians, we remain motivated and committed to delivering the highest in individualized care to our clients. Our dream is that someday nutrition and prevention medicine will be accessible to all as the cornerstone of healthcare in this country. This book is a step in that direction.

Contents

Introduction

It's quite likely that the number one reason you picked up this book is because you're looking for the right diet, the best diet to create the best YOU. How you arrived at this book might reveal a lot. Maybe you've taken advice from friends, colleagues at the office or experts on daytime TV that you need to eat this way or that. Maybe you've done your research and found science offers many, often-conflicting answers. Then there's the food pyramid, or triangle, or plate or whatever. Maybe you have a library of books, each with a very convincing argument for delivering the perfect diet. Maybe you've tried cuisines from more exotic cultures than your own. Maybe ethical food, or local food, is important to you. So how do you do it? How do you make sense of it all? At the end of the day why can't someone just clear it up for you, tell you what to eat and make the confusion go away?

The answer may surprise you. The answer may disappoint you. The answer may be so simple that it leaves you wanting. Or, as we hope, it may empower you. Before I share the answer I'll suggest that until you picked up this book most of the information you believe about what diet works best for you has come from unqualified sources. In that vein, we may not even able to recommend the best diet for you. You have to ask yourself, "why am I reading this book, then?"

So what's the answer? If no one is qualified to tell you, what does that leave? Surprising to many, it means that YOU are the most qualified to design the perfect diet for YOU. It means that YOU will be the one who solves the puzzle that delivers abundant health. It means that there may be truth to every diet out there but it will only work for you, if it works for YOU.

So after that little bit some people may decide to put this book back and that's fine. It doesn't mean we're going to tell you a different story just so we can sell a few more books. We recognize that telling you that you'll have to do some work isn't a sexy sell. Having to design your diet certainly doesn't seem as easy or enticing as the "other guys" program that promises: "you can eat whatever you want, get quick results and never have to do anything different." I can only offer that our office is full of the "now-wiser" survivors of those "get-healthy-quick" schemes. Our hope is that we will be able to save you from the metabolic damage that these programs create in exchange for white-knuckles, willpower fatigue, fleeting results, frustration, ultimate failure and self-esteem crush that you'll experience.

For a moment let's take a look at the most prevalent take on dieting today - the calorie model. You eat less and exercise more. You might think that diets are all different but oftentimes, they're actually just repackaged and rebranded variations on this model. In short the calorie model can be considered a math problem. The belief is that if you consume fewer calories than your body needs during a day you will lose weight as your body burns up the necessary calories from its own reserves, ideally from fat. It sounds pretty reasonable. It's clean and tight. It plays into our base needs for understanding and certainty. It sounds measurable and scientific. At first glance most wouldn't argue as its simple argument is almost non-negotiable. Everyone you know is familiar with the model so it's reassuring. Here's the problem. It fails in practice. The model is too simple for the magnificent YOU.

Here's why people stick to it though. In our recent history of diets and dieting most people have equated "getting healthy" to losing weight. The equation for health has been – you lose weight to get healthy (Decreasing Weight leads to Increasing Health). That's what your doctor, your friend, your spouse and your television are telling you, "Eat fewer calories and exercise a bit, then lose a little weight and you'll be healthy.

In marketing terms this idea is something that has "legs and life" in it. These are concepts or stories or whatever that survive the test of time, regardless of whether they're the best ideas or in some cases whether they're indeed true. It's called "stickiness". "Milk's got calcium, don't you know?" "Got milk?" "Milk is good for your bones." Milk is not nearly the best source of calcium but most everyone you know would rank it as a top source. So back to the calorie model for health, it's a very sticky concept. It's simple. It's easy to understand and by touting some certainty, it's kind of hard to argue with. It's backed by some science so I won't argue it's entirely wrong. The problem is that it's incomplete. Most of the story is missing.

Stickiness doesn't mean that it will work in practice. In fact, we find, the equation for health runs almost in reverse and delivers results that are much more in line with what most people actually want went they think about health. As I mentioned, getting healthy involves far more than just weight. More appropriately, your weight is simply under the umbrella of getting healthy. But regarding excess weight, what's proven in practice is that as you achieve greater health, you lose weight (Increasing Health leads to Decreasing Weight).

What you need to quickly take away is that simply losing weight does not mean you're healthier. In fact, most programs to lose weight actually leave you less healthy. But also, if you've made some dietary changes and you're not losing weight, you're not likely getting healthier. So, if you've made changes in your diet and lifestyle before that you were expecting to help you lose weight but you didn't, then your plan was likely wrong for YOU, perhaps altogether or perhaps just at that time in your life. In our new approach to health this is not a failure; it's a piece of the puzzle.

Now I need you to consider that your health is determined by far more than your weight. We've just been so focused on weight that we've lost the grasp of so much more. Consider this, we have a cross section of our clients that would be ideal on the cover of any fitness or self-fulfillment magazine in the country. They're fit, they're attractive; they're successful, but they're also unhealthy. At home at night or behind closed doors they may struggle with depression, anxiety, binge eating, hormonal issues, skin problems, digestive complaints, fatigue and on. So rarely do I meet someone that looks like the cover of a magazine that's also thriving in health. I don't have the skill with writing required for driving home this message so I can only hope that you can take this giant step with me. It's only through years of practice that I have managed to completely embrace this fault in our vanity and recognize that looking healthy in no way ensures being healthy. And with the broad and sweeping desire to look good over feel good, it's far more prevalent than most would ever consider.

I can imagine now that we're only a few pages into the book, you might be more confused than before you started. You're likely sticking around because I struck enough cords with you that you're willing to give this idea a chance. That's all we want. We have enough experience to know that a chance is often all we get and then people want to see results before they take in too much of our talk. I appreciate and understand so you're likely in just the right spot to begin.

We are going to take you on this journey of finding what works for YOU. It is a process that starts with discovering some unique principles and requires some commitment and awareness on your part. But don't feel overwhelmed by the idea of self-evaluation and experimentation. We lay out all the steps for you as you discover what your unique body needs. We will walk you through everything from how much water YOUR body needs to what form of exercise is best for YOU. Through questionnaires, a look at genetics and experimentation, you'll gather the pieces to solve the puzzle that of your unique health and discover the health you desire. Whether you're suffering from a chronic health condition, want to optimize your current level of health, or simply seeking a way through the web of health mis-information, the steps in this book will bring you to a new level of wellness - a level that can only be achieved by assembling the pieces of your unique health puzzle.

Section 1: Set Your Table

Your CHARGE

One of the most profound shifts you can make with regards to your health is to become your own health detective, a Health Private Investigator perhaps.

Simply put, your health is yours and your results are yours. You need to experience your health with an inquiring mind and without bias. This is no small task, especially the part about "without bias".

I can't tell you how much I loved the days when Snackwell's was considered healthy by all the latest research. I ignored how I felt because my taste buds were happy, and many experts suggested that these were the way to go. It was too good to be true. I was listening outside my body because I liked what I was hearing, but my body was telling a different story. We have a favorite, if unprofessional, saying around the office, "How's it workin' for you?" Well, the Snackwell's weren't working for me.

So, to begin becoming your personal health P.I., you need a system for tracking and making sense of how your diet and lifestyle affect you. Appropriately named the Metabolic CHARGE Journal,* this system is a daily routine that helps identify metabolic dysfunction. Greater swings or imbalance in these markers reflect a greater deficit in metabolic performance. The impact of this deficit may not entirely make sense- yet, so I simply ask you to start it and know that it should make sense soon.

CHARGE
> Cravings
> Hunger
> Attitude/Mood
> Rest/Sleep
> Gut/Digestion
> Energy

We're not focusing on details like calories, or grams of protein and carbs, here. The message is not to obsess about food. What you're looking to do is record what you eat across a day and begin to correlate your foods with your moods, energy, digestion, cravings, etc.- A lot of information can be uncovered from looking at what you eat daily (and across a week or more). More importantly, this exercise is about how YOU feel when you eat what you eat.

Your UP:

Begin to listen to your body. When you learn its language, you will begin to understand what works for you and what doesn't. Listening to your body is a skill that must be practiced but delivers tremendous reward when you do.

1. Metabolic CHARGE Journal:* Complete this health routine for at least three days, with ideal being at least one week. It's your first step in really listening to how food might affect YOU. You can maintain this routine beyond the first week, or anytime you want, as research shows it's actually one of the most effective health routines ever designed for anything from weight loss and arthritis- to-acne and depression. Simply grab a pencil and journal your routine and how you feel.

2. Begin to slow down and become present at your meals. Bring your awareness to your foods and food choices. See what you can piece together about your eating habits.

2

Name: _____
Date: / /
Day:

METABOLIC
C.H.A.R.G.E

Breakfast			Time	C.H.A.R.G.E
Time:				
Drink:		Meds/Supps ☐		
Morning Snack				
Time:				
Drink:		Meds/Supps ☐		
Lunch				
Time:				
Drink:		Meds/Supps ☐		
Afternoon Snack				
Time:				
Drink:		Meds/Supps ☐		
Dinner				
Time:				
Drink:		Meds/Supps ☐		
Evening Snack				
Time:				
Drink:		Meds/Supps ☐		
Time	Any Significant Daily Activities			

Record notable physical/mental feelings and timing
C: yes/no? when? for what?
H: Yes/no? when?
A: predominate mood during different times of day
R: how long? how well? times awake? Time for you?
G: notable GI signs or symptoms? when?
E: 1-10, rate through day? Quality?

Cravings   Hunger   Attitude/Mood   Rest/Sleep   Gut/Digestion   Energy

Clean Food

So I guess it's fair to ask, "What are Clean Foods?"

My concept of clean foods starts, essentially, with unprocessed whole foods, and ideally, local and organic.

An important aspect of Clean Food not raised by others requires that it "burns clean" in your body. A Clean Food works for you not against you. You metabolize it efficiently. It leaves you feeling clean, light and sharp. Your hair, skin, nails, energy radiate. Clean foods simply work for YOU.

This is where the <u>Metabolic CHARGE Journal</u>* becomes an essential tool. Here's the point: Some otherwise healthy foods may not work for your unique body and you need to identify them. This is important to grasp and requires that you learn your body's "symptoms language". Ask yourself, "Okay, how's it working for me?"

Foods that are not working well for you... we call them reactive or inflammatory foods. Really ANY food could be reactive for someone, but the most COMMON reactive foods are called the Sensitive 7.

Here they are: Wheat/gluten, Dairy, Corn, Soy, Egg, Peanut and Sugar. (If there were an 8th group, it would be the Nightshade family of foods - potatoes, tomatoes, eggplant, peppers, etc.).

This is a common joke in the Naturopathic Community,

Doctor: "Hi there, how are you? Would you please write down on this sheet of paper, your favorite foods and the foods you eat most often?"

Client: "Okay." (client composes the list) "Here you go."

Doctor: "Hmmm... I see." "Okay" (doctor hand the sheet back to the client) "Now here's a list of foods I want you to eliminate for the next 3 weeks."

Client: "You're kidding, right?"

Without boring you, I'll simply share that the foods we're sensitive to often fill out the list of our favorite foods. It's complicated and counterintuitive but it's real. This is a clue into reactive foods beyond the Sensitive 7 that may be unique to you.

Your UP:

"Clean up" your diet. Develop your personal awareness of foods that work for you. This process will be essential to developing your nutrition plan and taking your health into your own hands.

1. On your next shopping trip, if a product you're shopping for has a label, read it, and see if you can find any of the sensitive 7 ingredients. Look for them everywhere, even in the healthiest product you can think of... you're sure to be surprised.

[We are not asking you to eliminate these foods at this point, we are asking you to develop your awareness and discover where the Sensitive 7 hide. I can't give you a list of products - the products frequently change, but more importantly, you would be cheated of this insightful and essential experience.]

If you are interested, and you should be, about finding which foods your body thrives off of, look at our Clean UP Program* (formerly known as the 21 Day Metabolic Cleanse). We created it specifically with the Sensitive 7 in mind.

2. Make a list of your favorite foods, including foods you eat most often, maybe even add foods you consider comfort foods. Look at the list, break out your CHARGE journal and see if you can tie anything together.

Food Rules:

So if you haven't guessed already, I am a huge fan of all things Michael Pollan. He is a food writer with popular books like <u>Omnivore's Dilemma</u>, <u>In Defense of Food</u> and <u>Cooked</u>. I highly recommend them all! One of his shorter books is called <u>Food Rules</u>.

I love the simplicity of his approach to food. If you've read any of his books, you know the power of his sharp mind behind these simple food rules.

So, here's a sampling of some of my favorite Pollanism's from <u>Food Rules</u>:

You'll see... good nutrition can be SIMPLE.

1. Eat food

3. Avoid food products containing ingredients that no ordinary human would keep in the pantry

8. Avoid food products that make health claims

11. Avoid foods you see advertised on television

19. If it came from a plant, eat it; if it was made in a plant, don't.

20. It's not food if it arrived through the window of your car

25. Eat your colors

39. Eat all the junk food you want as long as you cook it yourself

47. Eat when you are hungry, not when you are bored

57. Don't get your fuel from the same place your car does

Look at your foods, your food choices and your food habits with a fresh perspective. This may require that you leave behind much of the nutrition myths you've been exposed to, daily, for years perhaps. For instance, #1 - eat food.... Few of us have ever considered doing otherwise but our grocery stores, full of aisles and aisles of "not-food", tell a different story about our eating habits.

Pollan's rules above offer a very broad but insightful nutrition perspective condensed into very simple bite-sized rules. For instance, "Eat Your Colors" simply reminds you to add colorful foods to your plate. Initially, you may be struck by how "brown and white" your diet has actually been. I won't bore you with how essential and powerful these "colors" are, but I also don't think that we need to consider it in more depth. If you "Eat Your Colors", your body will take care of the rest. If you don't, your body will struggle.

Your UP:

1. Check out the complete list of <u>Food Rules</u>* by Michael Pollan. Try to honor the food rules as you go through your week. Be sure to explore your old patterns and beliefs about food and see whether they are worth keeping or simply keeping you back.

2. Eat food this week. Consider what you eat in terms of food and not-food categories. The lines will blur a bit but it's in the simple practice that you will find the great benefit. So, is what you're eating, really food?

3 Inspired by Pollan's simple rules, we came up with our own rule - The Hundred Year Rule. About 100 years ago was a time before the massive industrial food revolution took hold and changed the quality of our food supply. If you would have seen a certain food, over 100 years ago, it's probably a fine choice!

100-Year Guide

While we have to live in our modern world, we use the 100-year rule as a guide for making healthy food choices. Choose health. Live health. Enjoy health.

Simply consider your foods and ask, "Would this food have made sense 100 years ago?"

- Simply… did it exist 100 years ago?
- Would your Great Grandmother have eaten this food?
- Can you picture the food growing in nature?

- What kind of processing does it take for this food to make it to my plate?

100 years ago. This roughly represents a time before the widespread existence of processed foods and industrialized food practices. Over the years since, we've tried lots of interesting things with our foods. Without advancing any agendas, I will offer the oversimplified view that many of our foods have been manipulated to improve them by some measurement or along the various aspects of their growth, production, distribution, preservation, and ultimate appeal or value. It seems like good business, but along the way, we've essentially invented many new foods and food-like substances that are, at best, marginally foreign, and at worst, completely alien representations of their former selves.

Among other things, we did manage to create foods that never spoil, and now we can splice fish genes with corn. While we could marvel at these feats of technology, I will argue whole heartedly that these advances have not truly improved food, but have in fact, significantly diminished their health benefits, and even made some harmful. It is this invented and broadly accessible diet that is so central to the most common chronic diseases of our time.

The 100-Year rule is more about perspective than absolutes. We won't try to identify the one or two most negatively influential "advances," but instead must present that it's the interplay of the total burden that adds up.

Some 100-Year Rule Standouts

This is about perception, not perfection, so start with these. Do what makes sense to you and works in your life, or perhaps take these and go even farther.

9

Fruits and Veggies

Buy fresh, local and seasonal... traditionally preserved fruits and veggies... frozen veggies on hand as a backup.

- Fruits and vegetables were grown in vital soils, delivered fresh, locally, and seasonally after ripening on the plant.

- Preservation was primarily by natural fermentation, as we consumed a fair amount of fermented foods.

- Juices were made fresh (not from concentrate or frozen) with no enriching, additives or preservatives.

Fats and Oils

Avoid foods labeled low fat, lite, fat free, or similar. Avoid highly processed fats like canola, corn, soy, peanut, safflower and margarine. Avoid fat alternatives/substitutes. Bring butter (in moderation) back into the diet.

- Fats were found naturally in foods with no offerings of fat-free, low-fat, and such.

- These were high commodity components of food and were used sparingly but completely.

- Fats were "clean" - free from foreign chemical and toxin residues.

- Machine-processed vegetable oil concentrates (soy, corn, canola, safflower, etc.), hydrogenated fats, and fat substitutes did not exist.

Animal Proteins

Opt for local, organic, free-range, pasture-raised, hormone-free, and wild-caught (or any combination) eggs, fish, meats, and poultry.

- Meats were naturally hormone-free, free-roaming, organic and were not hyper-immunized.
- The mass-produced, industrial feedlot farms did not exist.
- Animals ate the natural foods they were accustomed to eating.
- Meats were higher commodity, and we did not eat them with every meal. Portions were likely smaller.
- We used and ate every part of the animal for its unique qualities and health benefits.

Breads and Grains

If you can tolerate wheat, choose a sourdough bread that has been traditionally made with naturally occurring yeast. All breads should be eaten in moderation. Opt for whole grains made from scratch and limit processed grain products.

- Breads were made without yeast or through traditionally fermented yeast starters. Commercial quick-rise yeasts did not exist.
- Grains were whole and unaltered except by stone grinding. Bleached, refined, instant, and enriched grains (and the products made from them) did not exist.
- Breads were made fresh without additives or preservatives.

- Crackers, cereals, and chips as we know them today, did not really exist.

Sugar and Sweeteners

Avoid processed sugars and opt for sorghum, coconut sugar, local honey, and maple syrup. Liquid stevia is an option for those with blood sugar issues.

Consume all forms of sugar in moderation.

- 100 years ago, we consumed about 10lbs. per person per year. Currently, we average about 140 pounds per person per year.
- The only concentrated forms of sugar available were Cane sugar, sorghum, honey, molasses, and maple syrup.
- Highly processed sweeteners like refined white sugar, corn syrup, agave, stevia, and other artificial sweeteners did not exist.

Herbs, Spices, Seasonings

Be creative and add these highly nutrient-dense seasonings in your cooking to enhance the benefits and flavor of your foods. Salts should be unrefined. Vinegars should be raw and unfiltered. Season foods yourself and avoid pre-seasoned foods.

Drinks

Drink water. Consume fresh, unprocessed drinks.

- Drinks were fresh and unprocessed.

- Room temperature was likely most common.
- Teas were a mainstay, including herbal, white, green and black.
- High fructose corn syrup did not exist.
- Fresh water was essential.

We worked hard, made food from fresh, local, seasonal, organic ingredients, and we ate everything in moderation. Take the time to consider the healthfulness of newer, nontraditional foods, as well as newer production practices like plastics, microwaves, irradiation, and such.

Grocery Overwhelm:

Grocery stores can be overwhelming, at least for me. There are seemingly miles of aisles of different products, varieties and brands. We're going to try to simplify it for you. While I can't take each and every one of you to the grocery store (although it would be so fun.) I can point you in the right direction by giving you our list.

People like certainty, so most commonly we aim for our staples and get out, rarely daring to venture into the unknown corners of the store. So, while our list will simplify what to look for, some may find it initially involves more change than we're ready for... and that's okay... we're looking for progress now, not perfection.

Clearly this program is going to be about finding what works for YOU. It's about uncovering your own UP. For now, we are setting the foundations with the Founder Foods list. From a solid foundation you can create the diet that works best for YOU. While a list is quite boring, aim to bring some adventure to the experience by exploring new foods or new preparation.

Your UP:

Develop your foundation. Realize that every component of every cell in your body is built from the foods that you consume and absorb and utilize. Even your thoughts and emotions ride on the backs of molecules drawn from your diet. Out of love for yourself, select wisely. We're seeking progress not perfection.

1. Grab our Founder Foods Grocery List* and begin to build your diet from these foundation foods. Read over the list. Highlight the things that sound good to you. Take note of the things that are unfamiliar and venture to get to know them. We put them on the list for a reason.

Founder Foods
Real Foods Guide

Veggies

✓	Arugula	✓	Burdock Root
✓	Asparagus (7*)	✓	Butternut Squash
✓	Avocado (3*)	✓	Cabbage (4*)
✓	Bamboo shoots	✓	Carrots
✓	Bean sprouts	✓	Cassava
✓	Beet greens	✓	Cauliflower
✓	Bell peppers (7!)	✓	Celery (4!)
✓	Broad beans	✓	Chayote squash
✓	Broccoli	✓	Cherry Tomatoes 11!,#)
✓	Brussels sprouts	✓	Chives

- ✓ Collard greens
- ✓ Coriander
- ✓ Corn (#)
- ✓ Cucumber (9!)
- ✓ Dandelion greens
- ✓ Eggplant (8*)
- ✓ Endive
- ✓ Fennel
- ✓ Garlic
- ✓ Ginger root
- ✓ Green beans
- ✓ Green onions
- ✓ Hearts of palm
- ✓ Jicama (raw)
- ✓ Jalapeno peppers
- ✓ Kale
- ✓ Kohlrabi
- ✓ Leeks
- ✓ Lettuce (14!)
- ✓ Mustard greens

- ✓ Mushrooms (13*)
- ✓ Olives
- ✓ Onions (1*)
- ✓ Parsley
- ✓ Potatoes (10!,#)
- ✓ Radishes
- ✓ Radicchio
- ✓ Red Cabbage
- ✓ Red Potatoes
- ✓ Rhubarb
- ✓ Snap peas (15!)
- ✓ Snow peas
- ✓ Shallots
- ✓ Spinach (6!)
- ✓ Swiss chard
- ✓ Tomatoes (#)
- ✓ Turnip greens
- ✓ Watercress
- ✓ Zucchini

High-fiber, Starchy Vegetables, Beans, Legumes

- ✓ Acorn Squash
- ✓ Butternut Squash
- ✓ Spaghetti Squash
- ✓ Summer Squash
- ✓ Winter Squash
- ✓ Artichokes
- ✓ Leeks
- ✓ Lima Beans

- ✓ Okra
- ✓ Pumpkin
- ✓ Sweet Potatoes (12*)
- ✓ Turnips
- ✓ Yams
- ✓ Legumes
- ✓ Black Beans
- ✓ Adzuki

15

- ✓ Buckwheat
- ✓ Chickpeas (Garbanzo)
- ✓ Cowpeas
- ✓ French Beans
- ✓ Great Northern Beans
- ✓ Kidney Beans
- ✓ Lentils
- ✓ Mung Beans
- ✓ Navy Beans
- ✓ Pinto Beans
- ✓ Split Peas
- ✓ White Beans
- ✓ Yellow Beans
- ✓ Beets
- ✓ Parsnips
- ✓ Tempeh
- ✓ Miso

Meat, Fish, Poultry (#)

- ✓ Poultry (turkey, chicken, duck, quail, etc) (O,HF,FR)
- ✓ Beef (O,HF,GF)
- ✓ Lamb/Goat
- ✓ Seafood/Shellfish (WC)
- ✓ Fish (WC)
- ✓ Wild-game (buffalo, venison, etc)
- ✓ Eggs (O,FR,HF)

Fabulous Fruits
Lower Hormone Impact (consume preferentially)

- ✓ Blackberry
- ✓ Blueberry (13!)
- ✓ Boysenberry
- ✓ Elderberry
- ✓ Gooseberry
- ✓ Loganberry
- ✓ Raspberry
- ✓ Strawberry (2!)

✓   Green Apple (1!)

Moderate Hormone Impact

✓   Cherry
✓   Cranberry
✓   Pears
✓   Fresh Apricot
✓   Fresh Fig
✓   Melons
✓   Orange
✓   Peach (5!)
✓   Grapefruit (10*)
✓   Prune (Pitted)

✓   Red Apple (1!)
✓   Plum
✓   Kiwi (9*)
✓   Lemons
✓   Lime
✓   Nectarine (8!)
✓   Tangerine
✓   Passion Fruit
✓   Persimmon
✓   Pomegranate

Higher Hormone Impact (consume less)

✓   Pineapple (2*)
✓   Grapes (3!)
✓   Watermelon (14*)
✓   Cantaloupe (11*)
✓   Mango (6*)
✓   Papaya (5*,#)

Grains / Breads

✓   Quinoa
✓   Basmati Rice
✓   Millet
✓   Oats

- ✓ Polenta
- ✓ Brown Rice
- ✓ Wild Rice
- ✓ Amaranth Whole Grain Sprouted Bread
- ✓ Whole Grain Sprouted Tortilla
- ✓ Sourdough (Traditionally Fermented)

Dairy (#)

- ✓ Cheese (R,O,HF,GF,W)
- ✓ Milk (O,GF,HF,W)
- ✓ Cottage Cheese (O,4% or better)
- ✓ Yogurt (O,U,W)
- ✓ Ghee/Butter (O,GF,HF)

Friendly Fats

- ✓ Sesame Oil (R,LH)
- ✓ Walnut Oil (O,HH)
- ✓ Extra Virgin Olive Oil (R,O,LH)
- ✓ Avocado Oil (R,HH)
- ✓ Almond Oil (O,HH)
- ✓ Macadamia Nut Oil (R,O,LH)
- ✓ Coconut Oil (R,O,HH)
- ✓ Palm Oil (R,HH,Sust.Harvested)
- ✓ Butter (O)
- ✓ Ghee (O,HH)

Drink to Your Health

- ✓ Herbal teas
- ✓ Green/Black Tea
- ✓ Almond Milk (U)
- ✓ Rice Milk (U)
- ✓ Coconut Milk (U)
- ✓ Water (Pure/filtered or sparkling)
- ✓ Chicken Broth (O,LS)
- ✓ Vegetable Broth (O,LS)
- ✓ Fresh Vegetable Juice
- ✓ Miso

Nuts / Seeds (Raw, organic, unsalted)

- ✓ Almonds
- ✓ Chia Seeds
- ✓ Flax Seeds
- ✓ Hazelnuts
- ✓ Hemp Seeds
- ✓ Pecans
- ✓ Pine Nuts
- ✓ Pumpkin Seeds
- ✓ Sesame Seeds
- ✓ Sunflower Seeds
- ✓ Walnuts
- ✓ Nut Butters (R,O,U)

Sea Veggies

- ✓ Arame
- ✓ Kombu
- ✓ Hijiki Seaweed
- ✓ Nori Seaweed

Seasonings / Condiments

- ✓ Lemon
- ✓ Lime
- ✓ Cayenne (Spicy Peppers)(12!)
- ✓ Celtic/Himalayan Sea Salt
- ✓ Garlic
- ✓ Mustard
- ✓ Tahini
- ✓ Herbs/Spices
- ✓ Apple Cider Vinegar
- ✓ Brown Rice Vinegar
- ✓ Balsamic Vinegar
- ✓ Ginger (Fresh or pickled)
- ✓ Honey (Local,R)
- ✓ Maple Syrup (R)
- ✓ Brown Rice Syrup
- ✓ Coconut Sugar
- ✓ Stevia (Liquid)
- ✓ Pure Cocoa Powder (U,64% or better)

Canned Foods Suggestions

- ✓ Artichokes
- ✓ Tomato Sauce
- ✓ Tomatoes (Whole)
- ✓ Beans (Can be hard to digest)
- ✓ Salmon (WC)
- ✓ Sardines
- ✓ Tuna (WC,Dolphin safe)

Frozen Foods

- ✓ Berries
- ✓ Fish (WC)
- ✓ Spinach
- ✓ Kale
- ✓ Mixed Veggies

DESCRIPTIVE KEY
Recommended Qualities

R ... Raw, unprocessed, unrefined
U ... Unsweetened
NH ... Do Not Heat
LH ... Only Low or No Heat
HH ... High Heat Stable
O ... Organic
HF ... Hormone-free
LS ... Low-sodium / Low-Salt
WC ... Wild Caught
GF ... Grass-fed
FR ... Free-Range
W ... Whole (Full Fat)

Pesticide Residues of Common Foods
* ... Clean, low pesticide: Number is the rank - 1 is the cleanest, yeah.
 ! ... High pesticide: Number is the rank - 1 is the worst, boo. Buy organic.

Of note:
… Caution… frequently genetically-modified (GMO)

Add your own notes

Section 1 Recap

So, this is the end of your first section!

To a great extent each section will build for the next. So, at the end of each section, you'll want to reflect on your "UP" that you're working on to be ready for the coming week.

Your UP:

1. We congratulated ourselves on taking this journey.
2. We are looking at foods a little differently, now. Using Pollan's Rules, the 100 Year Guide and the Founder Foods list, we're identifying real foods and changing our relationship with them.
3. We are developing awareness around how food affects us with our personal Metabolic CHARGE Journal*

*Resources and handouts for Charge UP can be found at: http://healthecoaching.com/charge-up-program/charge-up-additional-resources/

Section 2: Digestion

Dig Your Digestion

So this isn't everyone's favorite topic but it's easily one of ours... digestion. I get that it might not be something to scream about so here's a little joke I like.

"The only time it seems appropriate to scream 'I have DIARRHEA'...
is when you're playing scrabble... because it's worth a boatload of points." Zack Galifianakis

While many of us might consider what's on our plate, we tend to put our head in the sand when it comes to this next essential step in nutrition. In our office we have a little saying, "Your health is like a bee, if you ignore it, it will simply go away." So in our minds, it's time to give digestion some solid consideration. An overriding theme is that good nutrition isn't simply about what you eat; it's about what you eat, digest, absorb and utilize.

Some fascinating facts about your digestion and why we care so much about it.

~ 90% of your brain serotonin (your happy, peaceful, calm neurotransmitter) is found in your digestive tract.
~ 80% of your immune system is found in your digestive tract.
~ The average healthy person carries about 5 pounds of healthy bacteria in their gut.
~ There are more neurons in your gut than your brain.
~ The digestive tract has its own nervous system, separate from your spinal cord.
~ Your digestive tract is not just your stomach and intestines; it also includes your entire mucosal lining -

your sinuses, vaginal tract and bladder. It's all connected.

~ Every part of every cell in your eye, your liver, your blood, your skin and on comes from the food on your plate.

Digestive Symptoms affect almost every system of the body. Common (but not normal) symptoms of sub-optimal digestion (read sub-optimal overall health) are the obvious things like, reflux, diarrhea, constipation, gas/ bloat... but also headaches, allergies, chronic sinusitis, chronic bladder infections, vaginal yeast infections, post nasal drip, autoimmune disease, anxiety, depression and on.

So, having a healthy gut is not just about the absence of gas or reflux. Optimizing digestive health is KEY for everyone who wants to live a healthy and vibrant life.

We chose to focus on digestion 1st in this series because is the most critical component of optimal health.

Your UP:

Open your mind to the central role digestion plays in your health. Recognize that beyond oxygen and water, good food that's properly digested is the next most critical influencer of total health, affecting every system in your body. Consider that any symptom you experience in your mind or body may be driven by a digestive weakness.

1. Take a look at your Metabolic CHARGE Journal and see if you can find any relationships between physical or mental experience and the foods you ate. You may not find any, yet, but begin to take notes and piece together the clues. Like with a puzzle, start to put the pieces together and soon the picture will come clear.

Gut Health Essentials

So there are 3 Essential Factors for good digestive health. With them in line, you're in great shape; when they're not, you're headed for trouble... you may, in fact, already be there. If you're already there, the good news is that the digestive tract is very responsive to beneficial changes.

1. Clean food
2. Robust Digestive Enzyme Function
3. Healthy Balance of Good Gut Bacteria

We're going to focus on gut bacteria, first.

No one likes to think of the trillions of bacteria that line the inside of our digestive tracts, but this is where the magic happens. Bacterial cells outnumber your human cells by about 10 to 1 so they deserve a little love and respect. It's only beginning to be understood but it is increasingly likely that our "gut bacterial gene pool" exerts as great or more of an influence on our health as the genes we get from our parents.

In a simple sense the bacteria are responsible for breaking down the foods we eat as well as protecting us from outside invaders which could make us sick. Because we are constantly exposed to unhealthy bacteria, our healthy bacteria are constantly trying to keep the bad guys in check.

An interesting note: I'm not sure if you've considered this but our GI tract is essentially outside world... It's like a tube running right through us where the outside world comes into contact with the inside world. We need it to be a healthy barrier.

Poor food choices, toxins, antibiotics (and other meds), sugar and stress are constantly taking a toll on our good bacteria creating the right "terrain" for the bad to take hold. When we lose the balance, symptoms follow, and any system of the body could be affected.

Our goal is to keep the good guys around... in great number, diversity and strength. Probiotics are the good guys and prebiotics are essentially food for the good guys. Prebiotics feed probiotics and probiotics feed your digestive, nervous and endocrine system. A healthy gut has a vast array of pre and probiotics.

PREBIOTICS and PROBIOTICS*
Support for Intestinal Health

Probiotics are associated with various beneficial effects involving intestinal health. Probiotics have been shown to improve the symptoms of diarrhea, inflammatory bowel disease, food allergy, and lactose mal-absorption.

- Live, active, cultured yogurt
- Kefir
- Tempeh
- Traditionally Fermented Sauerkraut
- Kimchi
- Miso
- Kombucha
- Traditionally Fermented Sourdough
- Pickled Veggies

Prebiotics are non-digestible components of food that can improve intestinal health. They stimulate the growth and activity of beneficial bacteria in the colon.

- Onion
- Banana
- Asparagus
- Chicory Root
- Maple Syrup
- Barley
- Oats
- Garlic
- Jerusalem Artichokes
- Leeks
- Dandelion Greens
- Mushrooms
- Rye
- Tomato

Other foods that promote intestinal health include:

- Dietary Fiber
- Low heat-processed Whey Protein Powder (people with dairy issues can be sensitive to whey)
- Glutamine (amino acid) *too much glutamine can cause excitability in some people
- Green Tea
- Chamomile tea

Jerusalem Artichoke Recipes

The Jerusalem artichoke, otherwise known as a Sunchoke,

looks similar to ginger root. High in iron, potassium and thiamine, low-fat Sunchokes also contain inulin, an indigestible fiber, which feeds the healthy bacteria (lactobacilli) in the intestinal tract. For this reason, they are considered a pre-biotic food. People with diabetes can enjoy Sunchokes as a potato alternative due to their slow absorption by the body. They can help prevent sharp increases in blood sugar.

Choose smooth, clean, unblemished, firm tubers with a minimum of bumps. Just as with potatoes, they can be baked, boiled, steamed, fried, and stewed. The peels are perfectly edible. Suggested spices include cinnamon, nutmeg, cloves, onion, and garlic.

Roasted Jerusalem Artichokes	
Makes 4 servings	
4 cloves garlic, chopped 2 ½ tbsp. extra virgin olive oil 1 ½ pounds Jerusalem artichokes Kosher salt and freshly ground black pepper to taste 1 tablespoon chopped parsley	Preheat oven to 500 degrees. Put garlic and oil in microwave-safe dish. Cover with a paper towel and cook at half power for 2 minutes. Set aside. Cut Jerusalem artichokes into golf balls pieces. Put in a shallow roasting pan large enough to hold all in one layer comfortably. Strain out garlic from oil over the chokes. Add salt and pepper and toss. Cook about 20 minutes (tossing once or twice) or until tender.

Basic Cooked Jerusalem Artichokes
Makes 6 servings

Jerusalem artichokes Lightly salted water Fresh lemon juice Salt and pepper	To prepare Jerusalem artichokes, cook in boiling, lightly-salted water for 1/2 to 1 hour, covered, until soft. Add salt and pepper to taste. Sprinkle with lemon juice.

Quinoa Sunchoke Pilaf Salad
Makes 4 servings

½ cup quinoa 2 Tbsp. oil ½ cup chopped onion 1 ¼ cup vegetable (or chicken) broth ¾ cup chickpeas, cooked 1 cup chopped Sunchokes ½ cup peas, fresh or frozen ¼ tsp. pepper	Rinse quinoa in a tight-mesh strainer under cool running water to remove the bitter flavor. Heat the oil in a 2-quart saucepan over medium-high heat. Add the rinsed quinoa and cook, stirring, until it cracks and pops, about 3 to 5 minutes. Add the onion and cook, stirring, until the onion is soft. Add the vegetable broth and bring to a boil over high heat. Add the chickpeas, Sunchokes, peas, and pepper. Return to a boil; reduce heat and simmer, covered for 20 minutes. Fluff with a fork.

*Please note - although the foods listed in this handout do contain pre and probiotics, research has not yet determined what portion sizes are most effective for promoting intestinal health. Source: Montalto M, et al., Probiotics: history, definition, requirements and possible therapeutic applications. Ann Ital Med Int. 2002 Jul-Sep;17(3):157-65, www.samcooks.com & www.homecooking.about.com

Your UP:

Become better friends with your bacterial buddies. Choose one pre/probiotic rich food to add to your diet each day. Try to vary your choices and keep track of your CHARGE.

Feed the Fire

So now we're going to talk about our food demolition crew, the digestive enzymes that deconstruct our foods into absorbable nutrients. This is pretty huge, but shouldn't be too hard to wrap your head around.

Perhaps the imagery of "digestive fire" may help. Here we have the wood as food and the enzymes as fire. A strong fire burns efficiently and effectively. On the other hand, a weak, slow burn mostly just smokes, even fizzles. And, of course, the quality of the wood makes a big difference too.
The steps of processing foods into usable nutrients are incredibly complex, crucial for health but, thankfully, it's essentially automatic. Here's the thing: Automatic doesn't mean you can forget about it. But, who wants to think about it? I know I don't. What I mean is you can't overlook it. If you do, eventually your body will make it your priority as simmering GI issues boil over and become part of every meal you ever try to enjoy and for hours afterward. We're hoping to skip that non-essential "joy" in life.

Today, we're talking about digestive enzyme function because I could probably quickly name 100 extremely common health complaints that are related to poor enzyme function and the improper break-down of food. I hope it's okay, but for simplicity, we are considering HCL (stomach acid) and enzymes under the umbrella of digestive enzymes. We carry a formula for our clients that includes both HCL and enzymes called SimpleZyme.*

So we have clients in our office all the time with weak digestive fire. It's very common. Digestive enzymes can be depleted in the short term or long term and need to be restored regularly. Again, much of the restoration is automatic but we know that doesn't mean we can ignore it. Also as we age, we're at a bit of a loss, too, as normal enzyme function diminishes, naturally.

The good news is that fixing digestive enzyme function can be a "ten cent" cure. It can be fairly simple and the benefits can be extraordinary.

Here are some essential first steps to stoke your digestive fire:

~ In the morning, before breakfast, drink 8 oz. of room temperature water with either 1 tsp. of lemon or 1 tsp. of apple cider vinegar.
~ Eat bitter foods like kale, dandelion greens or other bitter greens at the start of a meal to stimulate the entire digestive tract.
~ Chew your food, slowly, completely.
~ Take time to relax when you eat. Slow your mind. Breath from your abdomen.
~ Marinate meats in acidic "dressing". The acid pre-digests the meat, releasing tremendous flavor, and tenderizing the meat and taking some burden off your digestive tract.
~ Adding an acid based dressing to your green vegetables also helps with digestibility as well as making the minerals more bio-available to your body. It is no mistake that salad dressings are made with vinegar or lemon bases
~ Avoid drinking a lot of water, or such, at the start of a meal as it dilutes stomach acid.

~ Avoid drinking cold beverages, particularly around meal times. The cold shuts down the digestive tract shunting blood from the area and suppressing enzyme function.

~ If you already have weak digestive fire, raw foods, meats, high fat foods may be difficult to digest. Limit consumption initially, incorporate the other steps above, then reintroduce slowly as you stoke your digestive fire.

FOOD ENZYMES: Nature's Smart Foods*

Enzymes: "enzymes are complex proteins that act as catalysts in almost every biochemical process that takes place in the body". ~ Sally Fallon, Nourishing Traditions

There are 3 Classes:

> **Metabolic**: Happen within cells – protect cells, fight off infection, keep the body in "check".
>
> **Digestive**: secreted from digestive organs like pancreas - break down food into nutrients the body can utilize for energy, growth and repair.
>
> **Food**: enzymes found in certain foods which enhance the body's own digestive process. These are Nature's Smart foods. They are nutrient dense and highly digestible!

Smart Foods (enzyme rich) to incorporate into the diet:

1. 1 serving of your favorite raw veggie each day
2. When eating dairy, choose raw dairy, the enzymes have not been destroyed by heat
3. Naturally fermented foods
4. Raw nuts and seeds
5. Pre-soaked nuts, grains and legumes

6. Kombucha
7. Umeboshi plums
8. Ceviche
9. Sprouts
10. Apple cider vinegar, red wine vinegar, balsamic vinegar, Ume plum vinegar
11. Exceptional plant foods noted for high enzyme content include extra virgin olive oil raw honey, grapes, figs and many tropical fruits including avocados, dates, bananas, papaya, pineapple, kiwi and mangos.

Cooking will destroy some enzymes, but will also enhance the digestibility and nutrient content of certain foods. You need a balance of cooked and raw foods. Do not overcook foods - opt for light steaming, slow cooking and avoid grilling, frying foods and charring meats - the slower and lower the heat, the more nutrient dense and digestible.

Altogether, if you know that you have weak digestive function. There's a ton that can be done to restore it. For instance, smart incorporation of supplemental HCL and Digestive Enzymes can work wonders to get the fire started.

Your UP:

Stoke your digestive fire.

1. Start your morning with either water and lemon or water and apple cider vinegar at least 3 days in a row. See what you notice.
2. Add some of Nature's Smart Foods to your diet daily.
3. Take time with your food. Eat meals. Stop. Sit. Enjoy.
4. Start adding acidic marinades to any meat or fish dishes.

Stress & Digestion

The word stress is thrown around so frequently it has lost its meaning. But the significantly negative influence is not lost on your body. With respect to digestion, chronic stress has a cumulative and hugely negative impact. Whereas our minds can filter stress, perhaps accept it or mitigate it in some way as part of life, our digestive tract simply obeys the signals it receives.

So here's the simple conflict between stress and digestion. Digestion is governed by the parasympathetic nervous system. This system is defined as "rest and digest" and is the absolute opposite of your stress response which is governed by your sympathetic nervous system, defined as "fight or flight". These two systems function automatically and their relationship could be likened to a see-saw. As one goes up, the other goes down.

With stress coursing through your veins, the organs involved in digestion simply can't function properly. In conveying the significance here, it's hard to find a touchstone that we can relate to. Digestion is essentially automatic and subconscious. I might, however, liken it to the role chronic or significant stress plays with insomnia as sleep requires the same parasympathetic activation. A restless and racing mind is the effect of the sympathetic nervous system blocking the parasympathetic from delivering us into deep, restorative and restful sleep. You might limp through the night with a few winks but all benefits of sound sleep were compromised. It is the same for your digestion, whether you have an intimate experience you can relate to or not.

Your UP:

Bring awareness to the effects of stress on your digestive

health. Become mindful, not mind-full, when you eat. Track your CHARGE

1. Slow down for your meals.
2. Develop a tool to slow you down before eating. It may be as simple as parking the car instead of eating while driving between "meetings". Perhaps make time to breathe from your abdomen (lower stomach) for a couple minutes at the start of a meal.

Digging Deeper:

Chronic digestive issues are something we see daily in practice. If you have been focused on diet for awhile, but not getting the results you want, we recommend getting a comprehensive digestive stool analysis. This is a functional stool test giving insight into how your digestive tract is working (or not working). If you have ever tried to choose a probiotic at health food store, you are likely to get a rapid headache. There are so many strains, dosages and seemingly different benefits touted on the bottles. How do you know what works for YOU? Getting a closer look at your gut bacteria, inflammation and enzymes via a Comprehensive Digestive Stool Analysis (GI Health Panel*) will give you that extra insight into the inner workings of your digestive tract.

Although food sensitivity testing is controversial, we utilize IgG/IgA Food Sensitivity Testing* frequently in practice. We agree that if food testing were 100% reliable, no one would have to try different dietary approaches. We would all get our blood drawn and eat from a list of foods, easy! I wish it were that easy, but unfortunately, food testing is only a guideline or roadmap. It can give valuable insight into foods up regulating the immune response and to foods you are simply eating too often and your body does not like. Food testing, in combination with tracking your Metabolic CHARGE and experimenting with foods, is a valuable part of finding which foods are working and not working for your body.

Ease The Burden:

Some of our culinary traditions have great history behind them. For instance, the parsley that adorns your fancy restaurant meal is a wonderful breath freshener for after you've eaten. It happens to look nice too, so... nice work.

Here's a more appropriate one for this point in our program (it also ties into Dig Your Digestion). Salads are traditionally eaten at the start of a meal because the greens trigger bitter receptors on the tongue. These stimuli tell your Vagus nerve to wake up the entire GI tract. For a sluggish digestion, it's kind of like "heads up, here comes the boss, get back to work."

If you've discovered you don't digest protein well (or fats, or complex carbs, really), you may want to wake up your bitter receptors. The easiest routine is to add bitter foods at the start of bigger/more complex meals. In the list you'll find a handful of spices but it could include just about any herb in your kitchen... so spice it up.

Bitter Foods: Artichoke, Arugula, Asparagus, Broccoli, Brussels Sprouts, Burdock, Cabbage, Chard, Chayote Squash, Chicory, Watercress, Cucumbers, Dandelion, Eggplant, Endive, Grapefruit, Green Apples, Kale, Lettuce, Leafy greens, Lime, Lemon, Melons, Mushrooms (many kinds), Olives, Radicchio, Spinach, Sunchoke, Tomatoes, Uncured Olives, Zucchini

Seasonings/Spices: Chocolate/cocoa, Cumin, Dill, Fenugreek, Saffron, Sesame Seeds, Turmeric, Vinegar

Drinks: Coffee, Gentian, Quinine, Chamomile tea

Another trick is to use acidic marinades to heavier meals. These usually have citrus, vinegar or a similar base and begin breaking down the tougher proteins and fats well before you start preparing dinner. This is a tasty trick that takes the responsibility off your digestive tract.

In a similar manner, slower and lower cooking breaks down tougher proteins, fats and complex carbohydrates so you don't have to.

Lastly, perhaps more for information purposes, you can supplement with HCL (or pancreatic enzymes like pepsin for protein), when appropriate, to support a sluggish GI. Supplementing HCL (hydrochloric acid) is like adding stomach acid when you have a meal. It is actually myth that people with acid reflux have too much stomach acid. In most cases, the opposite is true, the symptoms of acid reflux are a result of too little stomach acid. I know this sounds very counter intuitive and if you have ever had problems with reflux, you know taking an acid blocker, like Pepcid, can really help with the symptoms. However, if you are looking for the cause, the underlying issue is usually low stomach acid. When people have low stomach acid, they are not able to effectively breakdown their food and keep it moving down the GI tract. Food get stuck under the lower esophageal sphincter and pushes upward. The result, you feel acid come up into the esophagus. However, if you produced enough acid to begin with, food would not be stuck and would not come back up!

The main causes of low stomach acid:

1. Stress
2. Low digestive enzymes
3. Not enough healthy bacteria
4. Food sensitivities: I am 99.9% sure almost every case

of reflux has to do with a food sensitivity. Up to the date of publishing this book (knock on wood) we have never had a person finish our Cleanse program and still have GERD! Since our program eliminates the common food sensitivities, you can see where my assurance comes from.

How do you know if you have low stomach acid?

Review your basic screening labs. Ones you should be getting annually from your Primary care physician.

Protein, Albumin, Globulin and BUN should all be within mid-range of the normal values. Too low or too high, even within the normal ranges but skewed to high or low, could be pointing to low stomach acid

You can perform an HCL challenge test. This is a functional look at stomach acid secretion. It will give you a general idea. Do not do this test if you regularly take acid blockers or PPI's or if you have a history of gastritis or a diagnosed Ulcer.

I recommend only doing it with the supervision of a qualified practitioner.

HYDROCHLORIC ACID CHALLENGE PROCEDURE*
Its Action In The Body

Hydrochloric acid (HCl) is normally secreted by the stomach to enhance the breakdown and subsequent absorption of the food and nutrients that we consume. HCl also serves a protective function, killing various pathogenic microorganisms that might otherwise cause infection in the gastrointestinal tract.

SYMPTOMS OF DECREASED HYDROCHLORIC ACID SECRETION

People with low HCl (hypochlorhydria) or absent HCl (achlorhydria) may be asymptomatic, or more commonly, may experience symptoms of impaired digestive function including gas, bloating and excessive fullness after meals.

HYDROCHLORIC ACID SUPPLEMENTATION
If hydrochloric acid secretion is believed to be low, HCl tablets can be taken. They are usually taken in the form of "Betaine HCl". Hydrochloric acid supplementation is usually a very safe treatment when done under appropriate medical supervision.

PROCEDURE
1. On your start day, start with one tablet (usually 500-750mg) of hydrochloric acid, at the beginning of a regular, complex meal (Note: This means a full meal with a variety of macronutrients, not a snack.).
2. Monitor for any side effects such as a warming sensation, discomfort, gnawing pain or burning in the throat or stomach. If you experience any of these symptoms, drink a large glass of water, consider taking an antacid, if necessary, and report the findings to our office. If these side effect symptoms are not present, proceed to step 3.
3. Increase your dose by one tablet of hydrochloric acid at the beginning of each full meal (this would be two tablets for full meal #2, three for full meal #3 and four tablets for full meal #4). If you note any of the above side effects, discontinue the HCL Challenge. Do NOT continue to increase the number of tablets. Report the findings.
4. You have completed the challenge when you experience any of the side effects noted above or you

reach 4 tablets with a meal and experience no symptoms.
5. Report the outcome of your HCL Challenge by listing the number of tablets per meal at which you experienced any symptoms and the dose of HCL per tablet. If you were up to 4 tablets per meal with no symptoms, then report that finding.

Your UP:

1. Add bitters to your diet to support digestive function

2. Marinate your "heavier" meals, and try slower and lower cooking methods.

3. Slow down for meals. We talked about this previously but HCL production is limited by cortisol (stress) and sympathetic nervous system activity (rushing around).

Section 2 Recap

Your UP:

1. We tracked our digestive symptoms in our CHARGE and slowly incorporated all of the components of a healthy digestive tract into our daily life
2. We are looking closely at inflammatory foods: Eat Clean
3. We added pre and Probiotics to our diet
4. We are using food enzymes to stoke our digestive fire
5. We are supporting healthy HCL production
6. We are making it a priority to manage stress

Resources and handouts for Charge UP can be found at: http://healthecoaching.com/charge-up-program/charge-up-additional-resources/

Section 3: Break(Fast)

Breaking Your Fast

Now we are moving to Breakfast. Grandma always said it was the most important meal of the day, and of course, Grandma's right.

You might hear us say something like, *"You only need to eat a good breakfast, if you want to feel good today, otherwise don't worry about it."*

Perhaps surprisingly, but like most things in nutrition there's a lot going on with breakfast, the meal when you Break (your nightly) Fast. We'll aim to keep it simple and get you thinking about how to start your day right for a positive Metabolic CHARGE all day.

So here's one of the biggest parts of breakfast. It sets up the cascade of hormones that will govern your day. These hormone signals ultimately govern how your body acts across your day, week, month, year, even lifetime. So for starters, what you eat and when helps decide:

~ How sharp you'll be at 11AM
~ Whether you'll crash and/or be anxious between 2-4PM
~ Your moods and ability to cope with stress all day
~ How you'll sleep that night
~ How you'll wake the next morning.
~ How you manage your weight (under and over-weight)
~ Likelihood of a host of chronic diseases
~ So much more...

The perfect breakfast is somewhat elusive as it depends on

YOU but we hope to narrow in on it. What is clear is that you MUST eat protein with breakfast. High carb breakfasts (cereal, oatmeal, fruit, bread/pastries, soda, caramel macchiato) do not work for anyone... you will flunk our list above miserably... eventually if not already. This can be hard for some to get over... take your time if you have to, but get over it. You'll be glad you did and won't want to look back.

We find that individuals need different amounts of protein and carbohydrate at breakfast... this will even change for you across your lifetime.

Your UP:

Set up your metabolism for sustained energy, your mind for clarity and your emotions for resilience and balance... everyday.

1. Eat a Positive CHARGE Breakfast* (or create your own in a similar vain) within 1 hour of waking up. If you exercise in the morning, you can wait until after your session but then eat within 30 minutes of finishing.

2. Keep track of your Metabolic CHARGE as you make changes to your breakfast. Try to discern which breakfasts work for YOU and which ones don't.

POSITIVE CHARGE
BREAKFAST IDEAS

Take these or get inspired…

- Hard-boiled or soft-boiled egg with melon
- Greek yogurt topped with strawberries and walnuts

- String cheese stick, brazil nuts and melon
- Leftovers from dinner (i.e., protein, veggie and grain… NOT pasta and bread)
- Smoked Salmon, cream cheese and sliced cucumbers
- Bacon and blueberries
- Sausage and grapefruit
- Protein smoothie with blended berries
- Mary's gone crackers, almond butter, hard-boiled egg
- Cottage cheese with cut up veggies (cucumbers, bell peppers, avocado)
- Hummus on sprouted grain bread or with veggies
- Mashed avocado on sprouted grain bread with handful of almonds
- Canadian bacon on ½ sprouted grain English muffin with butter
- Quinoa topped with almonds, blueberries and coconut flakes (serve chilled or hot)
- Black beans on a sprouted tortilla topped with salsa, avocado and spinach

*Veggies at breakfast will increase antioxidants, fiber and nutrients in your diet and start your day in a positive, hormone-balancing way.

Simple Quiche

2 pasture raised eggs
50g organic cream
30g grated raw cheese
10g diced onion
½ clove garlic (minced)
13g organic spinach

Directions:
Sautee onion and garlic together until onion is soft.
Whisk eggs, add cream, and pour into a greased ramekin dish.
Add cheese, onion, garlic and spinach.
Bake at 350 until top is browned.

**This quiche freezes well. Take out and re-heat for a quick, protein rich breakfast.

Breakfast, Not Your Thing

"Eat breakfast like a Queen, lunch like a princess, and dinner like a pauper." **Chinese Proverb (translated)**

So, this week, we're talking about the most important meal of your day. We're trying to convince you it's worth your time to make it a priority in your health, but the truth is that many of us simply don't have any appetite in the morning.

We need to tackle this issue. There are several mechanisms that can be at play here, but largely, "morning hunger" is a sign of a strong metabolism and quality sleep.

Regarding sleep, when we don't get restful sleep, the production of melatonin and leptin is altered, simultaneously leaving us groggy and without appetite. Elevated leptin suppresses appetite.

Regarding metabolism, the morning is a delicate time for blood sugar control. In this case, the absence of an appetite may reflect that adequate blood sugar is present but due to an undesirable excess of cycling cortisol. We lack the signals to eat food but not because of a robust metabolism but rather from a fragile one.

There's one last reason that we can't overlook - caffeine. Simply put, it's an appetite suppressant.

Whether it's poor sleep, poor blood sugar control, too much coffee or something else, later on in the day the rebound effect is, you guessed it, increased appetite, lost blood sugar control and CRAVINGS! Our hormones are a mess and we're along for the ride.

So, the question is, "Are you hungry in the morning and, if not, why?"

Your UP:

Stoke the digestive fire in the morning.

1. Re-visit the CHARGE journal, paying close attention to your mornings - what is your story? Too much coffee? Poor sleep? Morning stress?

Break(fast) experiment

As you know, this week we're playing around with the most important meal of the day. We'll give you the tools but this process will likely extend beyond this week as you find the routine that works for you.

Maybe tomorrow, maybe the next day, maybe even next week, I want you to add an experiment. You see, we find that some people can really only have protein for breakfast with no carbs. "Why" can be fairly complicated, so with a nod to keeping it simple for now, we just want you to see how it works for you.

[Please indulge me as I get out my soapbox for a moment] Here in the United States... a lot of our "breakfast foods" are a really bad idea for breakfast. Cultures around the world enjoy meals like beans and rice with egg, fish and rice, soups, chicken and veggies. Broadly, we're a convenience culture that likes the short-lived pleasures of sweet carbs in the morning. We reviewed this a couple days ago but I can't overstate the havoc it plays with your mind, body and emotions... it's time to ditch the "breakfast foods" for breakfast.

Your UP:

See how carbs affect your day.

1. For the next 3 days, skip the carbs (breads/pastries, orange juice, sugar in your coffee/tea, etc) and have only protein within 1 hour of waking. A couple hours later, you can have some carbs with protein (i.e., apple and almond butter) as a mid morning snack, if necessary.

2. Track your Metabolic CHARGE*

Protein choices: eggs (if tolerated), clean meats (think leftover from dinner: meat/ veggies), quality protein powder mixed with water or unsweetened almond or coconut milk, nuts or seeds

Digging Deeper: Quality Protein Powder

Turns out protein powders are quite controversial. Some say they are too processed and should not be eaten at all and those who do recommend protein powder cannot seem to decide on which kind. Protein powder is processed, of course, you can't pick it from a tree or grind it from a seed, but it still has many health benefits. Whey protein, for those who tolerate dairy, and many do not, is a good option as long as it is cold processed. Once whey protein has been heated, it loses most of its health benefits, in particular, its antioxidant properties. If your whey protein is super inexpensive or has a muscle bound partially naked man on the label, it is likely a heated form of whey and you should skip it! We like protein powders with a vast array of nutrients. Why take a separate multi vitamin when you can get it with your shake. Be sure to check for quality nutrient forms by reviewing our MAD DOC video with wallet guide.* We also like pea based proteins for those who have more food sensitivities. On our Clean UP Program,* we use a clean pea based protein, with all the good quality nutrient forms, called MetaMeal Pro*. I am 100% convinced that using this protein powder is a key reason why people are easily able to kick their sugar habit on the cleanse. For our Tighten UP Program,* we used a cold grass-fed whey protein powder that helps reduce cravings called CocoaCrave Pro.*

Coffee Talk:

One day the media tells you coffee is the ultimate health food and the next day, we're supposed to avoid coffee like the plague. So what's the deal?

Does it increase or decrease cancer risk...does it prevent or cause heart disease? Does it lower or decrease blood sugar? How about Alzheimer's? Dementia? Anxiety?

Here's why we're confused... there are studies to support benefits and risks in all of the above. "Well, how can that be?"... we have to wonder.

The confusion and controversy stems from how differently we all metabolize coffee. We have variations in our genetic makeup that dictate whether it's bad for us, neutral or even a health food.

Despite how we think we feel on coffee, it's not an indicator of which effect it has on our health. Without genetic testing, we simply have no idea whether our morning jolt is truly a friend or foe.

Regardless of the genetics involved, here are some insights for you morning ritual that you should incorporate.

~ Coffee really needs to be with a protein and/or a fat.
~ Add, organic full fat milk, butter or coconut oil (or all three) to your coffee to keep the blood sugar stable.
~ Eat breakfast with your coffee, unless you are going straight to workout.
~ Opt for organically grown coffee.
~ Don't have coffee after around 12pm. (Takes average of 6-10 hours to process the caffeine in one cup)
~ Decaf is not a healthy alternative. (If you do drink it, opt for water-decaffeinated varieties)

Your UP:

1. Pick a few days and try quitting coffee. At least 5 days is best. You can still have caffeine in the form of green tea, black tea or yerba mate. But ditch the coffee altogether and notice how you feel... do you even miss it? We often recommend quitting it whenever you can't face the day without it. It's no longer working for you regardless of your genes.

Coffee: Dig Deeper

I am a big fan of getting genetic testing to look for your nutrient needs, your hormone pathways and your ability to detoxify. Genetic testing is affordable and although a new area of focus in relation to nutrition, it is a wealth of valuable information. Within this information is how you metabolize caffeine. The cost of the test is worth finding out that information along, especially if you love coffee like I do! For more information on Personalized Nutrition based on your

50

genes, visit <u>BadMTHFR.com</u>*

If You're Ready…Another Break(fast) experiment

So, I've got another challenge for you, but at this point it may be more of an idea to keep in your sights. We had to add this to the Breakfast week but don't let it confuse you as you're getting into your new breakfast routine. You'll want to try this when your metabolism is burning clean and you feel energetic and vibrant throughout your day. So when you're looking to take your health to the next level it may actually be skipping breakfast a few times per week.

The term for this popular practice is intermittent fasting and it is a way to dip into your fat stores to help regulate your blood sugar. Think about yourself as a pre-modern person, hunting and gathering. You likely didn't have access to food at every meal but your genetic body is prepared with reserves. More appropriate today, your body actually benefits greatly from the occasional rest.

Intermittent fasting can help you tap into your genetic potential. This is not about skipping meals and starving. It is about running on your own fuel and "exercising" those metabolic pathways while feeling balanced and energetic.

There aren't really clear protocols for this, but the idea is to prolong the overnight fast by not eating "breakfast" until late morning or lunch time. These intermittent fasts are essentially exceptions to your new routine of eating breakfast everyday and are designed for a well-nourished and balanced metabolism, not a fragile one.

Dr. John Berardi from Precision Nutrition has written some great blogs on the topic.

Dr. Michael Mosley has written a few books, like the Fast Diet, and has great resources on his website.

Your UP:

Take your well-oiled, clean-burning and efficient metabolism to the next level.

1. When the time is right, practice intermittent fasting. Listen to your body. Track your CHARGE to see if it works for you.

2. Eat a well-balanced, protein and veggie rich meal to break this extended fast. Your body is going to absorb nutrients from your first meal very readily, so make it a good one!

Section 3 Recap

1. We recognized the type of food we choose to eat first and when we choose to eat that food can greatly affect our overall health and definitely how we feel on a day to day basis.
2. We are committed to finding what works best for us: protein only, protein with some carb or skipping breakfast.

Resources and handouts for Charge UP can be found at: http://healthecoaching.com/charge-up-program/charge-up-additional-resources/

Section 4: Protein Perplexia

Protein: Where to Start
What usually happens when you're talking nutrition and you pick one of the macronutrients like protein, everyone around you becomes a "diet team" authority. "Go high protein, because...." "Get it from plants, because...." "Eat only lean meat..." "It's about the ratios..." "It causes X, Y, and Z." "It prevents X, Y, and Z."

Your macronutrient needs (protein, fat and carbohydrate), and nutrition in general, might as well be added to politics and religion as some of the most uncomfortable conversations to start at a cocktail party.

But, I ask you again to open your mind and challenge what you "know". With nutrition as with many things... you can't always believe everything thing you think.

So this week we're tackling "Protein Perplexia" - a complex, yet common, condition defined by conflict and confusion regarding the consumption of dietary protein.

First of all, as creatures of habit, we like certainty, and "diet teams" offer that. Secondly, we all have our struggle and story and certain positions either agree or conflict with them. Lastly, each diet team can dig up some research that seems to support their views. No great judgment here but confusion and conflict only seem inevitable.

With a nod to simplifying nutrition, there are a few things that are clear about protein from recent research. Of all the macronutrients protein is the most filling and most likely to control cravings, balance blood sugar and support ideal body weight.

More specifically, branched-chain amino acids (protein building blocks found primarily in meat, dairy and legumes), increase longevity based on their ability to support liver detoxification, maintain muscle mass, bolster the immune system, balance neurotransmitters and aid in healthy weight/fat loss.

Now again to simplify your life, but also buck conventional nutrition "wisdom", we're going to forego references to ideal daily protein intake calculations. Despite the certainty that we love, they're complicated to maintain, based on wobbly research, misguided in their approach to wellness and really you're too unique for "average" recommendations to work in the long run.

Your UP:

Respect your struggle and story, but keep it simple and get enough protein. How will you know when you have enough? Track your CHARGE... your experience will ultimately guide you. In light of the benefits of protein above, listen intently and the answer will come.

1. Grab our protein list and get familiar with foods high in protein and how they vary.
2. Eat protein within 1 hour of waking.
3. Have protein with every meal or snack.
4. Have a small amount of protein 1 hour before bed (especially important for people with insomnia).

Protein Content of Common Foods

Meats, Poultry, Fish (cooked)

Chicken Breast	3 oz.	26g
Turkey	3 oz.	25g
Canned Tuna (in water)	3 oz.	22g
Steak	3 oz.	25g
Hamburger	3 oz.	22g

Salmon	3 oz.	20g
Pork Chop	3 oz.	19g
Ham	3 oz.	18g
Fish (white)	3 oz.	17g
Crab	3 oz.	16g
Bison	3 oz.	18g
Venison	3 oz.	22g
Liver	3 oz.	17g
Shrimp	3 oz.	17g
Clam	3 oz.	22g

Beans and Legumes (cooked)

Kidney Beans	½ cup	8g
Garbanzo Beans	½ cup	7g
Lentils	½ cup	9g
Refried Beans	½ cup	8g
Black Beans	½ cup	8g
Split Peas	½ cup	8

Grains (cooked)

Amaranth	½ cup	5g
Barley	½ cup	4g
Buckwheat	½ cup	3g
Millet	½ cup	3g
Oats	½ cup	3g
Quinoa	½ cup	5g
Brown Rice	½ cup	3g
White Rice	½ cup	2g

Dairy, Egg

Whole egg	1	7g
Milk (cow or goat)	1 cup	8g
Cottage Cheese	½ cup	12g
Yogurt	6 oz.	9g

Greek Yogurt	6 oz.	17g
String Cheese	1 Strip	6g
Cream Cheese	1 oz.	3g
Hard Cheese	1 oz.	3g

Nuts, Seeds

Peanuts (dry roasted)	¼ cup	9g
Walnuts	¼ cup	4g
Pumpkin Seeds	¼ cup	9g
Sunflower Seeds	¼ cup	9g
Almonds	¼ cup	6g
Sesame Seeds	¼ cup	6g
Flax Seeds	2 Tbsp.	4g
Cashews	¼ cup	5g
Nut Butter	2 Tbsp.	8g

Non-dairy Alternatives

Almond Milk	1 cup	2g
Rice Milk	1 cup	1g
Coconut Milk	1 cup	6g

Soy foods

Firm tofu	4 oz.	13g
Tempeh	3 oz.	16g
Edamame	½ cup	11g
Miso Paste	2 Tbsp.	4g

Other

Hummus	2 Tbsp.	9g
Spirulina	1 Tsp.	6g
Whey Protein Powder	2 Tbsp.	18g
Pea Protein Powder	2 Tbsp.	15g

Brewer's Yeast	1 Tbsp.	3g

Should You Eat Meat?

So, should you eat meat and if so how much?

This has to be one of the greatest nutrition debates in recent memory. And I want to share my experience so you'll understand how I answer this question.

I'm a passionate gal and love everything about empowered living, smart fitness and clean nutrition. In my younger years I tried every diet I could find, convinced each time that I had found THE perfect diet, advocated aggressively for it, sneered at others that didn't agree... only to discover what seemed to be a better way sometime later. I was macrobiotic, vegan, was a Zoner, tried South Beach, ate raw, did Atkins, flexitarian, locavore, gluten-free, dairy-free, and many more people have never heard of. I wasn't flaky; I was simply fueled by passion and love new research.

Now, back to our question. My answer on the meat issue is "It's up to YOU, you're the expert on this one." Your perfect nutrition plan needs to meet the needs of your story and struggle, your psychological sensitivities AND your physiologic expression. I deeply believe that there is no one perfect diet but the best plan for you is the one that you can commit to, own, love, live with and see results from. So your answer to this question depends on HIWFY ("How's It Working For You?, pronounced "hiffy"). Is your HIWFY "iffy"?

In truth, in the same way I might treat a diabetic for Diabetes, I often treat vegans for veganism, Paleo's for Paleolithic eating. When they come to see me, something's not working anymore and we need to try some changes.

So in my practice I absolutely honor my client's individual struggles and stories but I suggest you consider your HIWFY and entertain a challenge. If ethical reasons are not at the root of your vegan/vegetarian diet, I say try adding some animal meat. If you're purely Paleo, I say cut back on the meat a bit. You get the picture... if you're "All-in" in one direction, try bringing some counter-balance.

For every "diet team" out there I can show you people that are failing miserably while others thrive... the same is true about meat. For just about every bit of research out there, I can show you equally good research that offers a variation or even the complete opposite. The reason: The success or failure of the diet, or the research... whether it's positive or negative, depends on people and we're all just so dang different.

You see, it's all about HIWFY - you have to balance personal preferences, metabolism, sensitivities, genetic makeup, and such with positive and maintainable RESULTS.**
Do You Need More Protein?

You have gotten used to eating protein as a cornerstone of your daily menu. Now let's dig a little deeper.

We left yesterday suggesting you work to discover the type and amount of protein that works for YOU.

Here's a little quiz... to help with your exploration. (These are simple guidelines that I have found work for my clients.)

- Are you blood type O?
- Are you a thin, high stress female?
- Do you crave sugar and carbohydrates frequently?
- Do you have trouble skipping meals without feeling

lightheaded, shaky or irritable?
- Do you have a family history of diabetes or alcoholism?
- Do you have a personal history of anemia (low iron or low B12)?
- If you know your genes, do you have SNP's for MTHFR, BCMO, FUT2, PEMT?
- Do you have thinning hair or brittle nails?

If you answered yes to any of the above questions, you probably need more protein in your diet... sometimes a lot more, sometimes just a little bit more, more often.

You Are What You Eat, Eats

Admittedly, this starts out geared more towards those who get their protein in the forms of meat, fish, dairy, eggs, etc... but its message is fairly universal (so be sure to read to the bottom).

So... "You are what you eat, eats"... that is to say whatever your foods were exposed to, you're now exposed to... whether it's an apple or a steak - whether it's stress, pesticides, hormones, drugs, GMO's or whatever.

We talk about clean foods a lot and sometimes perspective is all that is necessary but it's also more tangible. Clean meat (insert: fish, dairy, eggs, etc.), for instance, is at the very least meat from an animal that was raised in a natural, open, free-roaming environment, allowed to eat the same diet it would naturally eat in the wild, has not been given artificial growth hormones, steroids or antibiotics. Ideally these animals are living in smaller, local farms, and humanely-raised and slaughtered.

From the perspective of animal rights and environmental sustainability, this is all fairly sensible, but few recognize how greatly clean meats (and veggies) impact their health. We're going to refer you to some experts in the wild meat industry for you to check out their research - EatWild.com.*

Your UP:

Consider the impact your food's diet, lifestyle and environment has on the quality of protein and ultimately, your health.

1. Do some research this week and find out where you can get the cleanest meats. Check out www.EatWild.com for a local farm in your area. If you are in a big city or cannot find clean meats, consider ordering from US Wellness Meats.*

2. If meat does not agree with you or your beliefs (and I respect this), or you're adding more veggie proteins to your diet, your shift this week is to make sure you do not have the same vegetarian source of protein more that 2 days in a row. You need a wide range of amino acids from protein and variety is key to this.

I find that many people in my practice (women in particular) may not get enough clean animal-based protein. Make it a priority to find clean meats, fish, etc.... If "clean" is not an option for you, as a health care practitioner, I think the issue may be important enough for your health to supplement or replace with more vegetarian sources of protein.

A Red Flag with Protein

When I hear a client say meat or protein slows down their digestive tract, a red flag goes up. So, in fact what I hear is,

"My digestive tract is weakened."

We talked about some of this in the second week but this is a timely review. Stomach acid, which is found at the very top of the stomach, is responsible for the first part of protein digestion. If stomach acid production is not adequate, protein is not properly broken down and symptoms arise like acid reflux, indigestion, slowed digestion (fullness, constipation, bloat, even nausea and vomiting). Poor protein metabolism ultimately leads to any number of issues that we looked into earlier this week.

Your UP:

1. Here's a quick little functional screening exam you can do right now to see if you're digesting protein well? A yes to any of them may indicate an issue.

- Look at your nails - are any at all rough with vertical ridges?
- Is your hair thin/thinning and/or dull for what you expect from your hair type?
- Do you have digestive symptoms like reflux, bloat or constipation?
- Is stress a #1 issue in your life? (stress hormone - cortisol - depletes stomach acid production)

2. If you have a set of screening labs done in the past year, take a look at them.

- Protein, albumin, globulin and BUN should all be in the middle of the normal range.
- Do you crave carbs and sugars despite having a balance of protein and fats?

Section 4 Recap

1. We becoming aware of our protein intake and how protein affects our CHARGE.
2. We are assessing our protein needs and deciding if animal or plant based proteins are ideal for us.
3. We are committed to buying clean protein sources

Resources and handouts for Charge UP can be found at: http://healthecoaching.com/charge-up-program/charge-up-additional-resources/

Section 5: Fix Your Fat

Fat is Your Friend?
The topic this week is a big one and might make you uncomfortable. Even reading the word "fat" can elicit deep reactions.

Well, for certain, dietary fat is the most confusing, even controversial, of the macronutrients. In the US we have a fixation with fat by comparison to the rest of the world.

In the 1980's dietary fat was pegged as the cause of heart disease (by way of elevating cholesterol) based on some interesting, but ultimately flawed research. Regrettably, this association remains one of the stubbornest "truths" in nutrition.

In the years since we adopted this fat phobia we've become more obese and seen increases in heart disease, cancer and chronic health diseases across the board.

So, what is the deal with fats?

Here is the short of it:
1. Fat does NOT make you fat... it simply doesn't and in fact, without fats, the body cannot burn fat.
2. Dietary fat (the right kind) does NOT contribute to elevated cholesterol levels.
3. Every cell in your body is made from a bi-lipid (double fat) membrane. If you want healthy cells (you do), you need to supply the body with adequate fats.
4. The biochemical pathways which produce your hormones and maintain balance come from dietary fat. If you want healthy sex hormones which among other things keep you young,

lower inflammation and improve your memory and sex drive (who doesn't) you need fat.
5. Your brain is about 60% fat. Wow, right? (same for your entire nervous system).

Have you heard of the French Paradox? Well, it's really not much of a paradox at all but was coined in the early 90's because French behavior flew right in the face of the emerging fat-free paradigm.

Simply put... the French have far better heart health than most despite their deep appreciation for wine, cheese, red meat and other foods pegged as guilty in causing heart disease.

We'll tease this apart this week as we explore the re-emerging understanding of fats and their beneficial role in health. This may be one of the toughest weeks to wrap your head around and I respect that.

Your UP:

Reconsider what you know and what you think about fats. This week we'll help you figure out which fats to look for and which to avoid.

I realize some may not jump right in after one email on fats but, this week I'm going to ask you to commit to a few steps.

1. Go "full fat" (otherwise considered "normal") whenever you have the choice this week.
2. Skip the fat-free, low-fat, 1%, 2%, etc this week.
3. When you're ready to take this step for your health, go to the fridge, the pantry and wherever and ditch the fat-free/low-fat yogurts, milks and cheeses, salad dressings, margarine, butter substitutes (including the "healthy ones" like Earth balance), egg substitutes, and all other manipulations of fat you can find.

Fat For Thought

We wanted to share a little more fat "food for thought" before we go any farther. We have written quite a few blogs on the topic. Please go to our site and take a look at them.

I think you'll enjoy them. They help set the tone for this week and I hope that they'll help reframe fats in a better light.

Coconut Oil: Healthier Hype?

Coconut Oil: A hero, not a villain.
It wasn't long ago that coconut oil was vilified for its high saturated fat content. The public was made to believe this food would cause high cholesterol, clog the arteries and increase body fat.

The exciting and ever changing field of nutrition is now painting a very different picture of coconut oil. Coconut oil is actually a health promoting food! I frequently promote the use of coconut oil in my practice and here are the reasons why...

1. Coconut oil is a medium chain triglyceride. It is metabolized very differently than other fats in the body. It is quickly absorbed, provides quick energy and promotes healthy digestion.
2. Coconut oil has a very high heat point, meaning it will not change structure in the presence of heat. This is a great anti-aging benefit since we believe the oxidation of fatty acids leads to inflammation and inflammation leads to premature aging.
3. Every cell in our body is made of a bi-lipid fatty membrane. In order for those membranes to stay

healthy, they need a certain amount of healthy fats, and that includes the medium chain fat from coconut oil.

4. Medium chain fatty acids are a key component of mother's breast milk, a perfect food for growing healthy brain neurons.

5. It also works great topically, as a moisturizer and a make-up remover. Just like we have to pay attention to what we put into our bodies, we have to pay attention to what we put on our skin. I cannot think of a safer, more natural way to moisturize the skin than with coconut oil!

6. MCT oil is a concentrated source of medium-chain fatty acids from coconut. MCT oil is rapidly absorbed into the blood stream making it a quick source of energy. It enhances weight loss, energy production, brain health and immune function. We recommend MCT Oil* as a component to our Tighten Up in 10 Program.*

Never Eat Roasted Nuts Again!
Well, at least not roasted nuts from the store.

Ok, so it is not about the fats- right? We know this. It takes fat to make healthy brain cells. It takes fat to make hormones. It takes fat to burn fat. Our fat free, high sugar, processed food days are behind us.

When is fat not healthy? When it is oxidized. Fat in the presence of high heat–fat becomes oxidized and toxic.

This is one of the reasons we eat only raw nuts and seeds during the Clean UP Program.*

Now, I love the taste of roasted nuts and I believe they can be a healthy addition to the diet when you roast them yourself.

When you buy roasted nuts at the store–

1. They can be roasted with unhealthy oils like canola oil
2. After being roasted, they are exposed to oxygen by sitting around on the grocery shelf
3. They can be roasted with processed salt, which we want to avoid

Nuts are really healthy but when we buy roasted nuts and seeds from the grocery store we really don't know how they have been prepared and stored–are they really healthy anymore?

The solution is to roast your own nuts and seeds and this is how you do it.

Here is a basic recipe. Honestly, I don't do a lot of measuring and weighing in my kitchen. I am too busy and what is the worst that can happen?

Roasted Nuts Recipe
Use whatever spices you like. Experiment with different nuts and seeds.

Watch your nuts and seeds, carefully – they can quickly overcook (and we don't want burnt nuts right? Heat combined with fat– not our friends- right!)

Ingredients:

      1/2 tsp ground cumin
      1/2 tsp curry powder
      1/4 tsp of cayenne powder

1/4 tsp cinnamon
1/2 tsp chili powder
1/2 tsp garlic powder
1/4 tsp of ground ginger
1/4 tsp of ginger powder
2 Tbsp. of coconut oil
1 Tbsp. of Sea Salt (optional)
2 cups of raw almonds (try your other favorite nuts as well)
*oh and I actually made these with cinnamon and coconut sugar one day– what a treat!

Directions:
1. Preheat oven to 325

2. Mix spices in a bowl and set aside

3. Heat oil in a skillet over low heat. Add spices and simmer for 5 minutes.

4. Place nuts in a mixing bowl and pour spice/oil mixture over to coat

5. Spread on a baking sheet and bake for about 15 minutes. Shake the pan a few times while in the oven. Watch the nuts–they quickly become over cooked!

6. Toss the nuts with any leftover spice mixture at the bottom of the pan.

7. Sprinkle with sea salt and let cool. Store in airtight container.

If you have not done this before, you are in for a treat. You can season them to your liking, they are super simple and so delicious, I promise you will never buy roasted nuts again!

Recipe Adapted from The New Basics Cookbook by Rosso and Lukins.

Cholesterol - The Myth.

Nutrition never gets boring (thankfully!).

In our modern society, we tend to go all or nothing and we have done it again with cholesterol. Cholesterol by itself is not the villain. Quickly, let me run through some of the benefits of cholesterol.

Cholesterol:

o Carries vitamins through the blood stream into your tissues

o Allows the brain to form nerve synapses

o Is a powerful antioxidant

o Cholesterol produces sex steroid hormones like estrogen, progesterone, and testosterone

o Cholesterol helps fight infection (viral and bacterial)

o Helps produce Vitamin D

There is so much more to the cholesterol story that meets the eye. A few times a year, I am a health coach at large corporate health screening events and I see (in mass amounts) how many people are deathly afraid of their cholesterol numbers. All they can focus on is, "How low can I get my numbers?"

If you're not ready for my take on it, do your research and learn about cholesterol biochemistry... you will be surprised. Systemic inflammation and your breakdown of cholesterol types (information well beyond your HDL and LDL numbers), are much more important. And, to be certain, extremely low cholesterol numbers do not equal good health and in fact, increase mortality rates.

Don't take it from me- do your own research and take a few minutes to a CBS interview from 2014 called Heart of the Matter – a two part program dealing with statins, cholesterol and heart disease*

Pay close attention to the very end of the interview to see what REALLY prevents heart disease. They also mention my very favorite antioxidant coQ10.

If you want an ideal cholesterol ratio and want to minimize inflammation… here is your answer!

"Better Cholesterol" nutrition plan:

o   Eat a healthy diet with plenty of vegetables. Avoid processed foods and buy whole foods whenever possible.
o   Food Sensitivities lead to inflammation. Find out if you are reacting to any foods in your diet.
o   Exercise regularly. Resistance training and interval training (mixed with yoga of course!) are ideal.
o   Don't smoke.
o   Manage stress in your life and take time for relaxation (massage, meditation, facials, yoga, Migun beds, saunas).
o   Detox Regularly. There is evidence that heart disease (and other chronic illnesses) are caused or exacerbated by an accumulation of heavy metals and other toxins in your body.

Digging Deeper: Cholesterol

If you have been part of the conventional medical model for years or have a family history of cardiovascular issues, you may be acutely interested in and aware of your cholesterol levels and probably afraid of eating fats in the diet. Not only is the correlation between high cholesterol and cardiovascular events quite controversial, there historical way of looking at cholesterol levels is outdated. If your doctor is looking only at total, LDL and HDL ("bad" and "good") cholesterol, then you do not have a complete picture of risk. It is important to look further at the breakdown of your cholesterol levels, called lipid sub-fractions along with inflammatory markers. Spectracell and Berkley labs offers some detailed lipid panels. It is also important to look at your genetics when it comes to fat metabolism, diabetes risk and potential to form clots. We also like to look at fatty acid panels to see what types of dietary fats a person needs and how well they are converting their fats. This can be done via a fatty acid test called the Holman Test.*

Additionally, time and time again we see, if you need to lower your cholesterol numbers, lowering carbohydrates and sugars in the diet will help almost every time!

Your UP:

1. Try roasting your own nuts and seeds this week.

2. If you don't have some already, pick up some organic coconut oil and begin to experiment cooking with it. It's also great for the skin as a moisturizer and sunblock. For the gals, it makes a wonderful eye makeup remover.

Fats: The Good, The Bad and The Processed

So, what really makes a fat healthy or unhealthy?

First, as more of a perspective than an absolute, healthy oils are the ones we've used traditionally, for centuries. A very general rule of thumb is whether you could squeeze or press the oil manually, or render it out with normal cooking, i.e. coconut oil, olive oil, grass-fed meat fat.

- New methods of high heat extraction, chemical extraction and high pressure extraction have increased production of lesser quality, lower cost oils with fewer if any health benefits, and in many cases, increased costs to health.

Second, you have to weigh quality of the fat. This can be a bit elusive to discern but it's perhaps the most important component. Quality is based on a few factors, requires both broad and specific consideration and varies with the fat source.

- For animal sources, healthy fats come from animals fed their natural diet in their natural environment. So, genetically modified corn-fed, hyper-immunized feed-lot cows, don't provide ideal butter, milk, or meat fat.
- For both animal and vegetable fats you need to weigh the unnatural production and manufacturing methods like pesticide use, hormone use, hydrogenation, homogenization, extraction methods (described above) and other artificial manipulation.
- If there were one thing I could almost universally say you should buy organic, it would be products that are high in fat. Many of the nasty practices used to get products to market involve chemicals that are fat soluble. In these products the chemicals can concentrate in the fats that you ultimately consume.

Third, you need to consider changes to the fat that occur in processing, cooking, and storage.

- Trans-fats, which are on the do not eat list, occur when the fats are exposed to higher heat than they can handle, high pressure, hydrogenation and other unnatural processing.

- Rancidity occurs for many of the same reasons but also due to sun, air and heat exposure. Fats have varying amounts of antioxidants that prevent or slow oxidation but when depleted due to exposure to sun, air, or heat, the oil will turn rancid and is no longer considered healthful.

- Heat plays a significant role in the healthfulness of a fat. Oils have varying heat points beyond which otherwise healthy fats can turn bad. Heat point must be considered when cooking with fats or preparing foods with high fat content.

This list puts processed foods almost universally on the do not consume list. You can imagine there's a spectrum or gradation when you consider best, better, worse and worst fats.

The Big "Healthy Fat" Myth

The Great "con" oil:
Olive oil comes from olives, peanut oil from peanuts, sunflower oil from sunflower seeds, etc.... Where does canola oil come from?

I'm so glad you asked.

Canola oil is a vegetable oil that has seeped into our food supply in a big way and managed to get the reputation as a healthy fat for its content of omega-3 fats. You'll find it everywhere in "healthy" versions of everyday processed foods. So... I strongly disagree with the health claims. (Hello, Thesaurus? Give me a stronger, more emphatic way to say "strongly".)

Many health experts (essentially "whistle blowers") cleverly refer to it is as CONola or CASHola (referring to the agri-/big-business profits made from this oil). While I am not radical and I don't chase down conspiracy theories too much, I do believe this one has succeeded in deceiving much of the health industry. I'm willing to stand at odds with the majority regarding this controversial oil because it doesn't add up

I think this highly processed vegetable oil should be avoided and here's the simple version why. The simple issue at hand is that this oil, from a rapeseed, goes through an extremely high heat, solvent extraction process. We talked about this yesterday, but the process destroys any potential benefit from the oil.

The larger problem is that you'll find it EVERYWHERE! Why? Because it's cheap and carries a wonderful reputation

Your UP:

Quit the Con-ola. Or at least, limit it in your diet.

1. Over the next week, read labels and start to notice how many foods contain canola oil. I think you'll find it surprising.
2. Move away from the products containing Canola.

This includes pre-made deli foods from healthy stores. TRY to find a healthy mayo or salad dressing without this highly processed oil. Let us know what you find.

Toxic Fat

We've encouraged you to begin thinking about fats broadly, with a fresh perspective but now we're just going to give you some simple specifics.

Unsaturated Fats (PUFAs and MUFAs):

- From variety of foods, mostly plant sources
- Fluid or more fluid
- Great for cells
- Destroyed by heat

Saturated Fats

- From animal sources (coconut and palm are exception)
- Solid at room temperature
- Withstand heat very well

Trans Fats

- Almost entirely manufactured by hydrogenation of unsaturated fats
- Industrial, synthetic, processed fat created to increase shelf life of foods
- Very bad for cells
- Don't belong in anything you consume
- Toxic food which should be removed from our food supply and is banned in several countries.

Some specific facts about fats that need to be given due attention.

- Oils should be treated with care so that they are not exposed to plastic, air, heat or light.
- Oils, particularly unsaturated fats should be stored in dark glass containers away from sunlight and used for low temp. cooking and salad dressings
- Fats used for medium and low temp cooking should

be of the saturated variety.
- High heat cooking is fun for a barbecue now and again, but you should limit it if fats are involved. Say NO to fried foods.
- Oils and fats that are no good for you include: oils made from GMO grains, margarine, trans fats, corn oil, canola oil, cottonseed oil, peanut, soy, and "vegetable oil"

Your UP:

Think about your fats like you would think about heirloom tomatoes from the market.... treat them with care-- they are fragile. Remember healthy fats create healthy cells... damaged fats create damaged cells.

1. Here's our breakdown of fats. Yes, Some, and No - Oils and Fats* Be mindful of which can endure cooking (and at what temperatures) and which can't.

Fats and Oils

YES

Grass-fed Butter	Avocado Oil
Grass-fed Ghee	Almond Oil
Grass-fed Meat Fat	Walnut Oil
Wild-Caught Fish Oils	Hazelnut Oil
Coconut Oil	Palm Oil
MCT Oils	Sesame Seed Oil
Extra Virgin Olive Oil	Macadamia Nut Oil
Cocoa Butter	

SOME

Pastured Bacon Fat	Safflower Oil
Grain-fed Butter	Sunflower Oil
Grain-fed Ghee	Lard
Grain-fed Meat Fat	Tallow
Duck Fat	Flax Oil
Goose Fat	Farm-raised Fish Fat
Chicken Fat	

NO

Canola Oil	Soy Oil
Corn Oil	"Vegetable" Oil
Cottonseed Oil	Margarine
Peanut Oil	Oils from GMO grains

Digging Deeper: Fats:

Occasionally you will find people who do not respond well to more fats in the diet. We think there is a genetic component, the APOE genotype. This is on the genes associated with Alzheimer's disease and increased cardiovascular issues. I think everyone should know their APOE genotype to help individualize their dietary needs. The most comprehensive way to look at this gene in combination with many other nutritionally related genes is to order a complete genetic panel at www.23andMe.com*

One Thing to Always Buy Organic

This could almost be considered a public service announcement. It's a bit heavy but it opens the door to a large concern that I think we MUST consider.

So... we mentioned this earlier in the week but fats (animal and vegetable) concentrate fat-soluble chemicals. And today, our environment is significantly more "synthetic" and "chemical" than just 50 or 100 years ago.

Here's a small glimpse of what we're up against. The overwhelming majority of our foods are now exposed to numerous chemicals in production and manufacturing. We have synthetic medications (hormones, antibiotics, etc), treatments for lawns and bugs, cleaning supplies and many other chemicals cycling in our environment. These chemicals can take years, even decades to degrade. They end up in our air, our water, our soil and ultimately in the foods we consume.

We're among the first generations that need to consider this stuff but we HAVE to. We have to take steps to protect our most valued personal asset - our health. And, if you have children (or dependents) you need to protect theirs for them. These chemicals are not benign; individually, some can cause devastating health problems and collectively we can only imagine far worse.

Now, back to the importance of their fat soluble nature. If you consume significant amounts of "dirty" fats, you can expect that your body will keep and store the chemicals. We don't eliminate fat-soluble substances very well. Storing them is perhaps a protective mechanism to keep these chemicals from cycling around your body but you're not protected. They will damage the fats in your body. Remember, your brain is 60% fat... essentially the same for your nerves. Every cell in your body is encompassed in a double-fat layer.

Finishing Fats
So, if there were one thing you'd buy organic... it'd be your primary sources of fat.

And, on that note... peanut butter... peanuts are one of the most highly sprayed crops. They readily grow mold, which is why so many people react to peanuts and why they require so much pesticide use. Here we have a high fat food, we spray it with tons of pesticide, blend it up to make peanut butter and then make our kids their favorite sandwich. Their brains are fragile and don't need the extra chemical insults. Go for peanut butter that has organic peanuts and nothing else.

So we flew through fats this week. It's such a big topic and we only had a week to cover it but we definitely broke 'em down. We tried to dispel some big fat myths, clarify some fat confusion and reframe this important macronutrient in a better, smarter and useful way.

Today is a day the day when we look back at what we covered and make sure we're caught up. Clearly, it will take longer than a week to get this down but now you have the tools to be your own expert.

- Healthy fats do not make you fat.
- Healthy fats do not contribute to bad cholesterol... it's about better not lower cholesterol.
- Your body needs fat to thrive.
- Healthy fats make healthy cells... choose wisely and handle them with care.
- Damaged fats make damaged cells... take care with heat, light and air.
- Say no to trans fats and rancid fats.
- Say NO to "foreign oil" - industrially processed and manufactured, dirty fats, low fat, etc....
- Organic is ideal when choosing your fats.
- Fats have different heat thresholds... be mindful and don't exceed them.
- Don't fall for the CON-ola.

Section 5 Recap

1. We are changing our perspective on fats and recognizing the role healthy fats have in our body
2. We are incorporating full fat products and avoiding processed "healthy" oils

Resources and handouts for Charge UP can be found at: http://healthecoaching.com/charge-up-program/charge-up-additional-resources/

Section 6: Your Sweet Spot for Carbs

Sugar: The Other Addictive White Substance
So this week, we're figuring out carbs. We're going to address the different kinds of carbohydrates this week but first we're going to talk a bit about sugar as a catch-all for simple carbohydrates. When we're talking about carbs and health, it's simple carbs that are generally most critical.

Ahhhh, sugar. Oh, how we love it! We love it so much that we have trouble saying no to it.

Let me ask you something. Have you ever decided that you are going to "turn the corner" and quit sugar for good, only to find yourself at the end of a row of Oreo cookies within a few days? Maybe it's not Oreos but you can probably identify... you find yourself asking, why? Why? Or maybe you've moved past the questions and just settled into the guilt and blame for your lack of willpower.

Here's the good news... and bad, really. We are genetically programed to want carbohydrates and sugars. If we did not have a built in receptors for sugar and a strong desire to consume it, we would never have survived as a species. We are deeply programmed (mentally and physically) to want, to need, to demand and to find sugar. So, it's not your fault.

Craving sugar is an instinct that begins with mother's breast milk but endures as a survival mechanism forever.

The physical and mental drives are deep. I liken resisting them to holding your breath. You can set your mind to holding it forever but at some point, rather quickly, your body says, "cute, that was fun... but I need oxygen and you're being silly" - deep breath in.

You see, sugar and carbs do a few essential things for us:

- they are the primary fuel for every cell in our body.
- they help produce serotonin (our happy, peaceful, "the world's a safe and wonderful place" neurotransmitter) - a serious coping mechanism.
- they bathe neurons in your brain thereby boosting brain function
- they stimulate the pleasure centers (dopamine) in the brain and body

Bottom line: Our need for sugar is not unlike an addiction. Sugar is essentially a drug: It's it's a highly refined concentrate with deep physical action and physical dependence develops quickly and easily. Here's the unique nature of it as a drug that makes it so problematic.

- It is easily accessible, abundantly available and cheap.
- Its a generally well accepted drug with socially approved norms for its frequent use.
- Kids love it and we love our kids. Our parents generally loved us the same way.
- We are hardwired to desire it from birth, unlike other drugs. It's in our nature.

Your UP:

Consider the powerful effects and pervasive nature of simple carbohydrates. Figure out if you're a sugar person.

You may already know but I find many have no idea how much they love sugar: Answer the questions below - are you one of my sugar people? Your answers are subtle, and less subtle, clues to your dependence on sugar.

1. Crave sweets, breads, pastas or alcohol?

2. Trouble skipping meals without feeling shaky or irritable?
3. Feel overly sluggish or foggy shortly after a meal high in carbs?
4. Alcoholism or Type 2 diabetes in the family?
5. Able to avoid eating sweets on a regular basis, but will never have them in the house b/c you know you will eat them?
6. Are you able to have a piece of bread, a square of chocolate or 1 cookie and feel satisfied or is it a trigger for wanting more?
7. Do you have carbohydrate or sugar cravings after a well-balanced meal?
8. Screening labs show triglycerides over 100 and/or fasting blood sugar over 95?
9. If you were asked to pick up trail mix at the store, would you find the kind with all the raisins, cranberry and other dried fruit? Similarly, if you were to make a smoothie, would you sneak in as many sweet fresh fruits as you could find?

Good Carbs / Bad Carbs

In my world there's much debate on this but are there good and bad carbs?

I want to walk you through the way I see it.

White sugar and a banana are both high in carbs. Clearly they're different sitting on your kitchen table but how about once they pass your teeth? Is there much difference? Does your body simply receive them both as sugar?

Yes, and no....

The sugar in each is still sugar but HOW your body receives it is different. Our banana has a better nutrient profile and higher fiber content which slows absorption of the sugar and aids in the sugar metabolism. It's a better option and not just marginally; it's a lot better.

So ultimately, the sugar content and overall complexity of the food plays an important role in how the sugar affects you.

Now, let's ask the same questions of table sugar and white rice (unnaturally, highly refined product). Is there much difference in HOW your body responds?

No.

White rice is milled rice that has had the husk, germ and bran removed. While the remaining rice is called a complex carbohydrate (starch), don't let it fool you. It exists as chains of simple sugars bonded together that are readily broken down into sugar.

HOW your body responds to white rice is not that different from the table sugar.

We'll go into this tomorrow but what we find is that many people are at a place with their health that it doesn't matter whether it's a banana, white rice or a teaspoon of sugar. It's all too much.

We'll continue to dig into why and aim to help you figure out what works for you.

But before we end we need to quickly talk about dietary fiber. Dietary fiber is a unique carbohydrate because, while it is composed of sugar molecules bonded together, the human digestive tract does not contain the enzymes to break them down for their use as energy.

Fiber is an excellent type of carbohydrate with profound health benefits. In our earlier example, the white rice has had all of its dietary fiber (and protein) removed leaving a poor quality food behind... ah, but it can stay on the shelf forever.

[It's important to remember but this is why calorie counting alone is a very poor health tool. Consider that 3 tsp. of sugar has the roughly the same number of calories and carbohydrates as 8 ounces of broccoli. Many popular health and weight loss programs would consider them equal.]

Your UP:

"Type of carbs" matters. Not all carbs are created equal.

Handling Carbs

Can you handle carbs? Some people can't.

Here is the thing-- some people can get all of the refined carbohydrates - cookies, cakes, breads and other sweets out of the diet and that's it. They feel on top of the world (their CHARGE fills up). While others crash from doing it right with just carbs from whole grains, fresh fruit or legumes.

Here we go again but per usual, it boils down to YOU and your metabolism. It comes down to your individual ability to breakdown sugar and the right hormone function that ensures the sugars get where they need to go, efficiently. If your metabolism is sluggish, inefficient or otherwise screwed up, you won't process them well and will feel like dirt.

So, we're going to see how you handle carbs but first let's get an idea how many carbs you're eating.

I don't love nutrition rules as you know but here's a starting point: I want almost everyone on less than 150g of carbohydrate per day. Even, under 100g per day.

While, I do not like to look at food as numbers, when we are tying to find your carb sweet spot, we have to do some math. Some people find they're right where they need to be (100g. or less) while others are shocked. I hope you find yours is eye opening, regardless.

Your UP:

Get real about your carbohydrate intake.

1. Over the next 3 days: Get an average idea of how many carbs you consume during a day... this includes all carbs, from rice and pasta to fruit and veggies. It should be unnecessary to say but, don't cheat yourself by eating differently.

Use an online program like www.cronometer.com* to track or look it up online carb-counter.net* and keep track of it in your folder. We are not getting crazy here; we just want a general idea. We're looking for net carbs which is Total Carbs per Serving minus Fiber times the number of Servings: Net Carbs = (TC - F) x S.

Find Your Sweet Spot

So what's your Sweet Spot for Carbs?

Your Sweet Spot for carbohydrate intake is the place where you're at your ideal weight (or on track to losing), you have balanced energy, a clear mind, sharp thinking and absolutely NO cravings for sugar or carbs.

Carb tolerance, like everything, is very individualized - some people do well on 100-150g, some can only handle fewer than 50g. Some have the luxury of doing fine on any amount. In this case, focus on better quality.

To make a point, you NEED adequate protein and fats in the diet but your carbohydrate needs vary.

Your sweet spot depends on YOU so we're back to our mantra - "discover, practice and master".

To find your sweet spot you will need to play with the Quantity, Quality, and Timing of your carbs and track your CHARGE.

Quantity:

Roughly, and for simplicity, one bite of
a starchy carbohydrates equals about 5g of carbs.

- Most will do well by eating 5-10 bites of carbohydrate per meal (some need more and some less)

However you decide to measure your carbs, we're considering net carbs.
Total Net Carbs = Total Carbs minus Fiber times the number of servings you ate. $NC=(TC-F)xS$

Quality:

The best kind of carbs are the clean (hypoallergenic) burning carbs:

- Rice (white or brown or wild)
- White, red or sweet potato
- Oats- gluten free

- Quinoa
- Bananas
- Plantains
- Yucca
- Fruits (overall should be limited to your dark berries)

Non-starchy vegetables are a free for all, yeah... so, you do not add to your daily carb count.

Timing:

- A great time to eat carbohydrates is within 1 hour after a workout - the body is sensitive to insulin at this time.
- Some people do well eating more carbs at breakfast and lunch and then very low carb at dinner.
- Others, particularly those with insomnia, will do well by having their carbs in the evening to help with sleep.
- Try to never eat carbs alone. Eat with an adequate amount of protein.

Your UP:

Find Your Sweet Spot

1. Experiment with Quantity, Quality and Timing. Track your CHARGE and find your unique Sweet Spot for Carbs. For perspective, ideally you're eating 3 meals per day and have a stable CHARGE all day. If you are used to eating snacks between meals or 5-6 mini-meals per day, keep that routine for now.

Surprising Place to Find Carbs

One of the most common myths for getting stable energy,

weight loss, and probably out of credit card debt is to eat protein bars as the ideal on-the-go snack.

I'm not sure if you noticed but protein bars are like sugar bombs with a little protein. By now, we know that sugar bombs are not good for us but how easily we're deceived by simple marketing. I mean it sure sounds like a protein bar would be mostly protein, right?

Here's the thing... to make cheap bars that people will eat... just add sugar. You'll likely find most of the bars that are easiest to find are not worth your time, money or health on this issue alone.

But here's our formula for picking the right carb and protein balance in your bars. I'm not sure about credit card debt but for stable moods and energy, hormone balance and the like, you'll want to make sure your bars pass the bar rule. And, per usual, you may be surprised how poorly your favorite bar does.

Here's the "secret" formula for choosing a bar - one that will keep you in your sweet spot:

Thanks to my friends and colleagues over at Metabolic Effect* for this:

Read the back label of your bar. Take Total Carbs per serving and subtract Fiber and Protein. You want the the per serving value to be less than 10. TC-F-P < 10 (Credit to Metabolic Effect for this formula.)

If it doesn't pass the test, it's not doing you any favors. We'll talk about this tomorrow but if it passes the test, the next step is to consider whether you need to be concerned about the other artificial or alternative sweeteners in it.

The Sweet and Unsweet Truth about Sweeteners

We want to share our Sweetener Guide with you. It covers 3 broad categories of sweeteners. Natural, Refined, and Artificial... note that some teeter between more than one category.

It's a fairly objective resource but by now you should be able to figure out which are better or worse, but here's a hint... finding a good sweetener is about much more than just calories. Go raw, go unrefined (or minimally processed), go natural.

Perhaps it's not conveyed in the Sweetener Guide but different sweeteners have significantly different physical effects... it's much more than the experience on your tongue. So, from my sweet perspective, (and theoretically of course) if I HAD TO CHOOSE between Coke (from Mexico), Coke (from the US) and Diet Coke... I'd go Coke from Mexico all the way. Why? Because among other things, it's made with sugar.

Occasionally. in the deep recesses of my mind I consider that someday, refined white sugar may make a comeback as a "health food". Forgive my cynicism but in contrast to the variety of contrived, unnatural and highly processed sweeteners available, white table sugar looks like a rock star. My body understands sugar; it's prepared to metabolize it correctly. Rant over.

So anyway, get to know your sweeteners. Venture out and try out new kinds. See if they affect your CHARGE differently. For me, one of my favorites is coconut sugar - very mild, with a good nutrient profile.

I will be sharing a fascinating story about a black market "underworld" related to one of the most universal, refined sweeteners that research suggests you're probably consuming near daily and might not even know it.

Digging Deeper: Sugar

Our goal with everyone is to get them off of all sugars. Having said that, sugar is everywhere and can be very difficult to avoid. We like raw, local, unfiltered honey, liquid stevia and xylitol, a sugar alcohol. Honey will increase blood glucose levels so it needs to be eaten in moderation, but it contains so many beneficial nutrients, we consider it a fairly healthy sugar for most people. Stevia and xylitol do not increase blood sugar levels and are good choices for diabetics, people needing to lose weight and sugar cravers. Even with these natural sweeteners, it is important to use them sparingly. Keeping the taste buds stimulated with sweet can cause increased sugar cravings for some people.

For optimal health and aging, please keep close track of your blood sugar levels. A yearly measurement of your fasting blood sugar on basic screening is not enough. Ask your primary care physician to run fasting blood sugar, fasting insulin and Hemoglobin A1c (HgbA1c). HgbA1c is a 3-month marker of blood sugar control and a very important marker of cellular aging. We will often recommend clients get a home monitor and test their blood sugars daily even if they are not pre-diabetic. This level of monitoring may sound extreme, but it gives you valuable information as to what foods are working for you and which ones are not.

When initially trying to get off sugar, we like using a formula with the amino acids 5-HTP and tyrosine in a balanced proportion called Crave Balance*. This supplies the brain with serotonin and dopamine. When these neurotransmitters are low, they cause us to crave sugar and alcohol. This is also a good formula for anxiety clients. Consult your health care provider if you are taking any psychiatric medications prior to

91

Your UP:

Learn the truth about sweeteners and make educated choices for your health.

1. Make better choices with your sweeteners. Get rid of sweeteners that offer no benefit or are simply bad for you.
2. Try out different sweeteners.

Now that you have seen the sweetener guide, for the most part, we want you to throw it away! Honestly, we want to get you to a place where you never crave sugars and could take them or leave them, except on a special occasion. When you have to have something sweet, you can make better choices with the sweetener guide. If you are changing your diet to reduce sugar, we like using small amounts of xylitol and stevia as you make your transition away from processed and artificial sweeteners.

Sweetener Guide*

Sugars and sweeteners are carbohydrates. Carbohydrates break down in the body into glucose (blood sugar) that supplies the body with the energy it requires to carry out activities and processes. Carbohydrates are the body's first choice for energy.

The best way to keep the body's mechanisms for regulating blood sugar working effectively is to eat a diet of 55–65% carbohydrates from whole grains, legumes, fruits, and vegetables. These types of carbohydrates are high in fiber. Dietary fiber slows the rate at which the stomach empties and absorbs carbohydrates, thus reducing after-meal blood sugar increases. Refined sugars lack fiber and therefore cause sharp increases in blood sugar.

There are three main groups of sweeteners: natural sweeteners, refined sugars, and artificial sweeteners.

Natural Sweeteners
Although most natural sweeteners can cause many of the same problems as refined sugars when consumed in excessive amounts, they are considered better alternatives since they retain many of their original vitamins and minerals.

Date sugar	Dried, ground dates. Contains folic acid.	Substitute 1:1 for white sugar. Add hot water to dissolve date sugar before using in batters. Use in combination with other sweeteners for baking.
Fruitsource (Brand name)	Granular or liquid product made from grape juice concentrate and whole-rice syrup. Glucose, fructose, and maltose.	Substitute 1¼ cup for 1 cup white sugar. Reduce salt 30% to 50%. Bake at 325° F to 350°F maximum.

Sucanat (Brand name)	Dried, organic sugar cane juice- minerals and molasses retained.	Can be substituted 1:1 for white or brown sugar in cooking.
Amasake	Made by fermenting sweet brown rice into a thick sweet liquid.	Use in puddings, cakes, pies. Can be used as warm or cold beverage. Refrigerate.
Barley Malt	Sweetener made by fermenting sweet brown rice into a thick sweet liquid.	Substitute 1 1/3 cups barley malt for 1 cup white sugar. Boil for 2-3 minutes before adding to recipe. Reduce liquid in recipe by ¼ cup. Purchase only 100% barley malt.
Blackstrap Molasses	Syrup remaining after third and final extraction of sugar from boiled juice of sugar cane or beets. Source of iron.	Can substitute molasses for brown sugar in recipes. Reduce liquids in recipes by ¼ cup per cup of molasses. Refrigerate.
Brown-rice syrup	Made by sprouting brown rice in water.	Good for cookies, crisps, granola, pies, and puddings. Substitute 1 1/3 cups for 1 cup white sugar. Reduce liquids by ¼ cup per cup rice syrup. Refrigerate.
Concentrated Fruit Sweetener	Commercial syrup made from peach, pineapple, pear, and other fruit juices that have been cooked down.	Use in all baked goods. Substitute 2/3 cup for 1 cup white sugar. Reduce liquid by 1/3 cup per cup of fruit sweetener. Refrigerate.

Honey	Flower nectar that is collected, modified, and concentrated by bees.	Use in all baked goods. Substitute ½ to ¾ cup honey for 1 cup white sugar. Reduce liquids in recipe by ¼ cup per 1 cup of honey. Reduce oven 25⁰ F and adjust baking time. Don't give honey to children under 2.
Maple syrup	Made from boiled sap of sugar maple trees. High in potassium and calcium.	Use in all baked goods. Substitute 2/3 to ¾ cup maple syrup for 1 cup white sugar. Reduce liquid in recipe by 3 tablespoons. Refrigerate.
Sorghum	Syrup-like sweetener made by concentrating juice of boiled sorghum (a relative of millet) stems.	Use in baked beans, granola, and puddings. Substitute ½ to ¾ cup sorghum for 1 cup white sugar. Reduce liquids by ¼ cup per cup white sugar. Refrigerate.
Other liquid sweeteners	Pureed dates, pureed banana, applesauce and apple butter, fruit juice, frozen fruit juice concentrate.	Amounts vary depending on recipe.
Stevia (ground leaves or stevioside)	Whole dried stevia leaves ground into fine powder. Stevioside is dry powder extracted from stevia leaves. Several hundred	Substitute 1 ½ to 2 teaspoons stevia leaves or ¼ teaspoon stevioside for 1-cup sugar in recipes. Reduce liquids to adjust.

	times sweeter than sugar.

Refined Sugars

Refined sugars supply the body with calories and energy, but have little nutritional value. The refining process strips sugar cane or sugar beets of their vitamins and minerals, leaving behind sucrose. Consuming large amounts of sucrose can lead to nutritional deficiencies, obesity, and tooth decay. The following refined sugars are best limited or eliminated from the diet:

Turbinado sugar ("Sugar in the Raw"): Light brown crystals separated from molasses in the first extraction. It is 95% sucrose.

White sugar: Refined turbinado sugar that has been further washed and whitened (everything from the cane or beet removed)- 99.9% sucrose.

Brown sugar: White sugar with molasses added- 96% sucrose.

Confectioner's sugar: White sugar pulverized to powder with added cornstarch.

Fructose: Highly refined fruit sugar that comes in liquid or crystal form. The liquid form is derived from corn syrup with enzymes added and then heated to separate fructose from glucose. Although this is a highly refined simple sugar with no nutrients, it is absorbed into the body rather slowly. It is also very sweet. Substitute 2/3 to 3/4 cup for 1 cup sugar, and decrease baking temperature by 25°.

Corn syrup: Highly refined sweetener made from corn, steamed and deodorized to produce the odorless, clear, tasteless, sweet syrup. It is found in many processed foods, including pancake syrup, candy, jelly, juice and soda.

Sugar alcohols: Sugar alcohols are specific types of carbohydrate which are not readily broken down by the digestive system and thus have very little effect on blood sugar. They are very sweet to the taste buds, are found naturally in some fruits and the body produces some sugar alcohols on its own. sorbitol, erythritol, mannitol and xylitol are some of the most common. Because of the additional benefits of preventing cavities and strengthening bone, we like xylitol as an alternative sweetener.

If you over consume sugar alcohols, you are likely to experience digestive issues like gas, bloat and diarrhea. For people with digestive symptoms already, sugar alcohols may not be the best choice.

Agave Nectar: This is a popular sweetener found in many different "health" foods. It has long been touted as a great substitute for refined sugar because it is high in minerals and does not spike blood sugar levels. In the past, it has always been marketed as a diabetic friendly sweetener. Unfortunately, this is too good to be true and agave nectar is actually worse for blood sugar control than sugar. Agave is very high in fructose (not glucose) so it does not register in the same way on the glucose scale as other sugars and carbohydrates. However, because it is so high in fructose, it spikes insulin levels and is difficult for the liver to process. It is a very POOR choice of sweetener.

References:
Cynthia Lair's, Feeding the Whole Family, 1998, Nutrition Handbook for Nursing Practice 1993, Staying Healthy with Nutrition, by Elson M. Haas, M.D. 1992, Whole Food Facts, by Evelyn Roehl 1996, and www.cspinet.org

The Dark World of Sweet Drugs

Would you believe that there's an underground international black market trade for US's favorite sweetener?

So the Carb section is ending and I wanted to close with a fascinating, scary, crazy reality regarding one of the most prevalent sweeteners, the world over. It's a story worthy of a sensational international espionage crime thriller.

We're talking about the sinister, corrupt, and high stakes trade of honey. Yup, just like we all suspected, the teddy bear shaped bottles had to be a cover for something evil.

Anyway, the US consumes an estimated 400 million pounds of honey annually with over 60% of it imported. It's estimated that over 3/4 of that honey is not what the bees made but is some adulterated variation or simply a syrup. According to the FDA it can't legally be sold as honey but the FDA apparently isn't equipped to monitor and manage this enormous issue. Reportedly, there is no way of telling if it's real honey or simply a syrup without looking at the pollen granules in the honey, under a microscope. These granules can also identify country of origin based on the profile of the pollen. Ahh... but our love for the ultra-filtered honey has required that we remove it all.

With historically high market prices for honey, there's significant money to be made if you can produce a lot cheaply and get it to the US... open the door for unsavory and eager producers. Honey from China has a reputation for being highly processed and adulterated and was banned by the US after it was regularly found to contain toxic chemicals, illegal animal antibiotics, excessive heavy metals and simply water (to increase volume production).

The Chinese still eager for their share of the market ultra-filters out the pollen and then launders it through a web of untraceable international buyers before delivering it to the US market.

I'm not quite the storyteller to give this tale its due drama and tension but I don't think it's a stretch to liken it to international drug smuggling.

I share this story because part of me is fascinated by it but the doctor in me feels the need to add perspective on the often intense influence that sweets have on our lives, our cultures, and our world.

Section 6 Recap

1. We looked at the ubiquitous nature of sugar in our culture. Big food industry knows how much we like it and how addictive it is.
2. We got real about our sugar intake, even from "healthy" sources like dried fruits and whole grains.
3. We started to track our intake, focus on protein and alternative sweeteners.

Resources and handouts for Charge UP can be found at: http://healthecoaching.com/charge-up-program/charge-up-additional-resources/

Section 7: Drink To Your Health

Foundations

More than 15 years ago, I read a book called, Your Body's Many Cries for Water* by Dr. Batmanghelidj. It's a fascinating read especially in light of this programs intention, establishing the foundations of health.

With every one of my clients I hammer home my thoughts about the foundations - clean air, clean water, clean food, movement and sunshine. For many it seems too simple. I might hear, "With all of the fancy things we're capable of in medicine and science, you're telling me I need breathe, drink, eat, and go for a walk?" You see, you can take the newest supplement, try the latest celebrity diet, or get a cutting edge nutrition profile test, but at the end of the day, if you don't set the foundations for health, you and your body will continue to limp around in search of better health.

Consider this - next to oxygen, water is the most essential "nutrient" we consume... just try going a couple days without hydrating. I think intellectually we get it; we recognize thirst. But, many have never considered hydration much more than a daily chore. Most have never truly grasped the level of influence it must have on our health and therefore have never recognized it as powerful medicine. Clean water IS absolutely powerful medicine.

The scientific literature has associated these common health conditions with dehydration.

- Migraines
- Headaches
- Fatigue
- Back pain
- Arthritic pain

- Asthma
- High blood pressure and low blood pressure
- Type 11 diabetes
- Colitis- inflammation of the large intestine
- Elevated cholesterol
- Acid reflux
- Constipation
- Mood disorders
- Cardiac Arrhythmia
- Muscle cramps
- Death

Put a different way, if you have any interest in improving mental and emotional clarity, decreasing or ending pain, preventing chronic disease, optimizing blood sugar, burning fat, and freedom from digestive distress - you have to stay hydrated.

Your UP:

Develop a greater respect for one of the most accessible, cheap, and powerful tools in medicine - hydration.

Read the following bullet points and track your water intake this week in relation to these signs. What do you think- are you hydrated? Of note: If you are chronically dehydrated, you can no longer count on your thirst mechanism to notify you - so you may need to drink because it's time, not because you're thirsty.

- Cracked or dry lips
- Sticky mouth
- Normal urine from a hydrated body is pale-yellow. If it is bright or darker yellow-- you are not optimally hydrated. Clear urine may be from over-hydration.
- Skin turgor test: grasp skin on the back of the hand with two fingers so that a "tent" forms. After a few

seconds, release the skin - it should bounce back immediately. If any tenting remains or it is slow to return to normal, this reflects significant dehydration.

Consider tracking your CHARGE on days when you're hydrated vs days you forget. See how dehydration affects you in the short-term.

Water: Controversial Basic Human Need - Part 1

I guess we can make a controversy out of anything but I think at the very least, it's worthy of a discussion. Part of the controversy with water is over how much we need.

What is clear is that water is a readily available and ideal fluid for hydration. How much you need, though, is the muddied part of the conversation. There is a lot that affects your total intake, personal needs, use and excretion.

Take these into consideration:

- You get water when you eat fresh, whole foods like veggies and fruit, drink herbal teas or soak in a bath.
- If you sweat a lot, are an avid exerciser, drink coffee (or other diuretics), soda (regular or diet) or eat a diet high in carbohydrates - you are decreasing your cellular hydration.
- Age plays a factor. The older we get, the less efficient we are at utilizing water. Chronic dehydration is a biomarker of aging.
- Body fat affects needs. The more body fat you have, the lower your ability to utilize water. Body fat is a buffer against cellular hydration.

This was only a brief glimpse but essentially each person has unique water needs. It even varies from day to day, from month to month, and as you age or your health changes.

Your UP:

Hydrate Your Life.
A general guide is to drink 1/2 of your body weight in ounces of water daily... So if you weigh 120 lbs., you would drink 60 ounces of water. Now this does not take into account all of the above-- food, exercise and body fat. But it is a good starting place for everyone.

This week- every morning- measure out 1/2 your body weight in ounces in the morning- so you know how much you need to be getting in throughout the day. Sip through the day, not all at one time.

Take note of your Metabolic CHARGE as the week goes on - what are you noticing?

Water: Controversial Basic Human Need - Part 2

We need water but our water isn't what it used to be. In the vein of creating a strong foundation, the quality of our water must support that foundation not undermine it.

Have you ever wondered how clean your tap water is? If so, have you done your research looking for a water filter? It's more than a little confusing, right?

So, first of all, water quality varies from region by region, state by state and city by city. When you have a moment check the Environmental Working Group's (EWG) website* for tap water reviews to see how your area scores. If not listed, you can try calling your local water company for testing results or some companies will test your water for a variety of different parameters.

The truth is that modern water concerns like chlorine, fluoride, solvents, pesticide runoff, pharmaceuticals, and on make a good water filter a necessity in every home. I wish it were different, but truthfully, few of us still have good clean water.

We advocate everyone get a water filter (or filters) in their home for drinking, cooking and bathing.

You need to do your own research and decide what type of filter will work best for you and your family - there are many options. We like <u>Aquasana water filters</u>*- they are inexpensive and great quality-- if finances allow, a whole house filter is ideal!

I can't skip over the bottled water trend so, despite the enticing marketing, bottled water is often a far worse choice than water on several levels and has the added environmental impact.

So, make some educated choices about how you hydrate.

Your UP:

Make sure your choice of water supports a healthy foundation.

1. Do your water research.
2. If you don't have a good water filter - plan for the investment in your health.
3. We recommend watching the movie Tapped*
4. For some common sense comedy relief, watch It Doesn't Make Sense to Buy Bottled Water (1 min.)*

More, Coffee Talk

Let me ask you something, "Is coffee good for you?"

With coffee it seems one day it's the ultimate health food and the next, you should never touch it. What's the deal?

I'll break down the cause for confusion. What research does show is that if you have a group of 100 people and you gave them all coffee, 50 of those people will find tremendous health benefit from the coffee:

• lowered cardiovascular disease risk factors
• improved blood sugar control
• cancer prevention

The other 50, however, will experience the exact opposite. Coffee will not be good for them at all!

The problem is that we don't know which 50 individuals will get which effect. The difference is in the way we metabolize coffee in the liver. It is a genetic difference and is independent of how coffee makes you feel or how much you like it. An important note: it's not just about the caffeine... it's coffee.

Digging Deeper: Coffee

These days with specialized testing we can actually get the genetic perspective and tell whether coffee is a health food or not for YOU (and so much more). We utilize genetic testing via 23andMe. Although the company no longer offers health information specifically, it does give access to your genetic information in its basic form called the raw data. The raw data can be plugged into various online app's and you can start to get a picture of your nutrient needs, neurotransmitters, hormone pathways and detoxification pathways, which brings us back to coffee. Via genetic testing you can find out how you metabolize coffee....is it a health food for you?

"Utilizing the raw data from genetic testing (from 23andMe) has allowed me to take individualized care to a whole new level. Along with a detailed intake, screening labs and genetic testing, we no longer have to make educated guesses at what someone needs to optimize their nutrition. We can now put all of the pieces of someone's unique puzzle together. These advancements are a gift to individualized and effective client care." ~ Dr. Sherri

Aside from genetics - here are some broader guidelines for whether coffee is working for you:

Ditch the coffee if...

1. You have issues with anxiety or insomnia-- yes for some people, if you are a slow coffee metabolizer, that 1 cup of coffee in the morning can prevent you from getting a good night's sleep.
2. You can't start the day without your coffee.
3. You have blood sugar issues - you can't skip a meal without feeling irritable and shaky.

Your UP:

Decide if coffee's working for you... or you're getting worked by it.

1. Experiment with stopping or reducing coffee this week: You can still get your caffeine fix from green or black tea, but see how you do without or by limiting coffee. Go slow if you have to as you may get headaches. Pay attention to your CHARGE.

Decaf coffee is not a suitable substitute-- the caffeine is usually removed by exposure of the beans to terrible solvents. If you must have decaf coffee, opt for a water-extracted decaf coffee in order to skip the toxins.

Juices, smoothies, teas, broths- oh my!

We have to recognize that there are many fluids that are ideal for hydration but mixing in some nutrient-dense selections can take our health to the next level without much, if any, effort. My favorite way is with homemade bone broth. It's rich in minerals, I think it should be a staple for anyone who is looking for extra nutrients that prevent aging, and support healthy collagen formation (think: skin tone, strong/shiny hair, healthy gut lining, strong/resilient bone and nimble joints).

Teas:
Never underestimate the power of herbal teas - subtle but powerful medicine we have been using since forever.

- Green tea (all varieties, matcha, jasmine), black tea, red tea, white tea and oolong
- Chamomile for nervous tension and sleep
- Red raspberry and nettle for hormone balance and minerals
- Peppermint tea for digestion
- Licorice root for modulating cortisol
- Thyme tea as a powerful antiviral
- Rosemary tea for mental clarity, and added energy
- You name it. There's probably a tea for every "kind of day" or condition you can imagine.

Juices:

I am not a huge fan of fruit juices across the board even made at home from fresh squeezed fruit (this should be considered a treat). I have to be a little picky but usually it's due to the sugar content in the final juice. Consider this, there's essentially the same sugar content in store bought orange juice as there is in your average can of soda. Juice wins by comparison of benefits but it's still a lot of sugar.

We recommend pomegranate juice--- but you only need 1/3 of a cup per day

Green juices can be great. Experiment with them. We don't recommend more than 1 cup per day. Beware of bottled juices sold as green juices. They're often just green sugar bombs.

Souping is the new juicing. Green juices are high in nutrients, but they lack the fiber content, which is why it is really important to avoid the juices with fruits in them. They will spike your blood sugar. Even better than juicing, is souping. Instead of extracting all of the juice from a vegetable, why not steam the veggies and then use a hand-blender to mash them up. Add a little sea salt and coconut or grass-fed butter and you have a high nutrient, fiber rich thick beverage. Soups and purees are easy to digest, increase hydration, and you can pack with herbs, spices and really max out the nutrients.

Smoothies are a great way to get lots of nutrients in one drink. Focus on lower sugar content fruits like frozen berries. Get creative with what you add: nut butters, spices, coconut flakes, dark cocoa nibs, use unsweetened liquids, dark green leafies, avocado, and so much more. And, as always, use your CHARGE. Simply because something should be healthy, doesn't mean it is for you.

We think it is important to add protein to your smoothie. Protein powders are controversial. If you are not sensitive to dairy, we recommend a cold processed, non-denatured whey protein from grass-fed cows. When whey protein is from factory farms and processed using heat (read cheap), you lose the health benefits of whey, including the immune support. We also like pea based protein for those who cannot do dairy. We recommend finding a protein that contains a full spectrum of nutrients. Why not power up your smoothie!

Digging Deeper:

Nutrients: On the topic of nutrients, we are very particular about the forms of vitamins you choose. Whether you are looking for a quality multi or a protein with quality nutrients, the forms matter. When we are using genetic panels to personalize a client's nutrition needs, we clearly see how some forms of nutrients like folic acid, could potentially be harmful. We created a wallet guide to help you choose high quality supplements.

There are a variety of ways to test for nutrient status. One of our favorite and easiest ways is to look at an Organic Acid Panel.* It requires a simple morning urine sample sent to the lab.

Are your supplements MAD DOC approved?*

Methyl...

> Look for methyl forms of B12 and Folic Acid. You want to look for the "methylcobalamin" form of B12 and the "methylfolate" form (or simply the word "folate") for folic acid. A product that contains these ingredients shows a greater degree of integrity in research and product design.
>
> ***Note: It can be extremely difficult to find an over-the-counter supplement that contains both of these forms. If you do find one, you can bet it is a great supplement. You know this company has done its research!
>
> ***At the very least, try to find a company that is at least using methylcobalamin and not cyanocobalamin.

Additives

Some additives are common in product formulation but look out for red flags - Hydrogenated oils, titanium dioxide, and natural flavors are a few examples.

Dyes

There's no reason for your supplement or multi-vitamin to be some fancy color. It's marketing. Extra money spent on marketing tends to mean that less money was spent on the product.

Difference

Your time, energy and money are spent on these vitamins and they should be making in a difference in the way you feel and in your labs. Too many people take a product because they read somewhere that they should take it. Well, we want to see you thrive when you take it.

Oxides

Look out for oxide forms of minerals. Red flag for a poor product. These forms are inexpensive and are not readily absorbed by the body so they will pass right through you. Common ones to avoid are zinc oxide, magnesium oxide and copper oxide.

***Oxides tend to have laxative effect so the one place where they might make sense is in a laxative.

Calcium Carbonate

Red flag for a poor product. This form of calcium is an inexpensive, very poorly absorbed form. We might consider it a "cosmetic" ingredient... it's listed on the outside of the bottle but the health benefits are not delivered by the inside of the bottle. Quick quality-control check… if you see this form of calcium, you can skip this product.

A few expanded notes:

MAD DOC will help you quickly rule out which products aren't worth your time or money. Unfortunately, it may not make life easier for you as you may quickly find that many of the offerings in your local store are not MAD DOC approved… not worth your time or money, broadly speaking. So, I recognize MAD DOC is kind of a mixed-offering. I wrestled with this as I created it but I had to get this information out. Simply put, it makes me mad that very poor products are being sold to you. And, I feel it's through awareness that we can begin to make change and we must demand better products. At the very least we, collectively, need to quit paying for poor quality products.

So, what do you do? You may or may not be aware that some supplements/products are only available through a qualified health care practitioner. These products are often referred to as professional or doctor-only product lines. In many instances these products far exceed the quality of more easily accessible products. Unfortunately, but perhaps reasonably, they do tend to be more expensive. Do your research and find reputable professional and/or non-professional products. Hopefully, MAD DOC will help you get started.

Your UP:

Variety is the spice of life... and health. Sneak in added nutrients anyway you can, especially when you hydrate.

1. Incorporate some green juices and herbal teas this week. Make teas hot or make a large batch and out in the fridge for cold green or herbal tea. If you need a little sweetener, add a

drop or two of liquid stevia.

2. Try roasting a whole chicken sometime soon and make a bone broth from the leftovers. Bone broths put store bought soup stocks to shame. Sip throughout the day, use as base for soups, or use for making any grains.

C's Blue Avocado Spin*
a.k.a… Charge UP Smoothie

This is an All-Star Smoothie with our clients and may soon be one of yours.
It's designed to get your motor running and keep it burning clean for hours.
Start with 8-12 ounces of unsweetened almond or coconut milk as your liquid base.

Add Ingredients:

> 1/2 scoop of <u>MetaMeal Pro</u>*
> 1 scoop of <u>MetaClean</u>*
> 1 Cup frozen blueberries
> 1 Cup fresh spinach, cleaned
> 1/8 avocado slice
> 1 Tbsp. raw cocoa nibs
> 1 Tbsp. chia seeds
> 1 tsp. cinnamon powder

Blend in your <u>Vitamix</u>* or other blender until smooth. Enjoy with a smile.

I guess the weird name of this smoothie may help you remember the ingredients
> C's – Chia, Cocoa, Cinnamon
> Blue – Blueberries

Avocado
Spin - Spinach

The Worst Diet Ever

I realize that this isn't relevant to everyone but we all need to hear it. I'm just going to come out and say it... quit the diet drinks. I'm talking about diet soda, diet teas, diet "whatever".

I have a quick story on why I feel this way. I had a client long ago that always comes to mind. He was an addict/alcoholic in recovery but the only relevance there was that he had successfully managed his addictions to crack cocaine, methamphetamines, alcohol and tobacco for a couple years. He was coming to see me because he couldn't get off the diet soda. His diet soda addiction was destroying his brain chemistry and mental health and it had begun to ruin his relationships with his wife, children, colleagues and friends. Please don't think that this only happens to people with "addictive personalities". Addiction to diet drinks is rampant.

Why are we so addicted to diet drinks?

Artificial sweeteners stimulate dopamine release in the brain (affecting our reward center). Yes, they actually change your brain chemistry in the same way as any of the other addictive mind-altering substances. But, mix the brain stimulation with a sweet taste and a caffeine boost, then market it as something good for you that delivers swimsuit model results... now, you have quite a troublesome combination.

Tips for getting off diet drinks:

- I guess number 1 would be to admit whether you have a problem. I'd say if you're drinking it, you probably do or you may soon.
- Doing this program - the healthier you become, the more nutrients you ingest from a clean diet, and the more balanced your metabolism is, the less your body will want toxic sweeteners.
- Soda water with frozen berries or flavored liquid stevia (they actually make cola and root beer flavors).
- Amino acids like glutamine, tyrosine, and tryptophan can help support the neurotransmitters in the brain. Natural production of beneficial neurotransmitters reduces the craving and seeking behaviors.
- Anything to stabilize blood sugar (remember what you learned in your sweet spot for carb week).
- We really like DopaBoost* by Designs For Health for getting people off diet drinks.
- Stepwise transition from diet to regular soda and then to juice or water or such can ease the process if you're struggling.

I think that you can take much of this to heart for any product containing artificial sweeteners. Recognize that products that play with brain chemicals are designed to induce craving and seeking behaviors as well as withdrawal effects.

Your UP:

Recognize that diet drinks are simply the result of great marketing for a product that's terrible for your health. Research has shown that they do not help with weight loss and several quality long-term studies have shown that actually increases weight gain. They are mind altering and, therefore, not to be taken lightly.

A Milk Mustache

All the beautiful celebrities with perfect skin, white teeth and slender figures... you would think the milk mustache is a MUST, if you want they have.

Don't be fooled. By now you know, it's just good marketing. And about the calcium, you can get more from your green leafy vegetables than a glass of milk.

However, a question to ask is, "Should I drink milk?". Like everything else in nutrition, it largely depends on you. It may be good for you; it may not. That's up to your genetic and metabolic make-up.

There are people on every side of the milk issue with deep and passionate beliefs but in my clinic with the responsibility for others' health in play, I don't have the luxury of their all-or-nothing conviction. My clients have managed to confirm as well as debunk nearly every side of the dairy issue so I am left with the objective view, that much of it depends on you. During our Clean UP Program, we walk clients through the process of eliminating the inflammatory foods, dairy being one of them. At the end of the 3 weeks, we add it back in a specific way so you can see if dairy is working for or against you. But, for certain there's a tremendous amount about dairy that is not dependent on you and must be considered before giving your body a chance to offer up its own opinion.

First, there is no reason you have to drink milk. So, if you never drink milk, don't worry - you're good. We don't need it. But, if you do drink milk, get in the know about your milk.

We have nostalgic memories of the days when milk was hand-delivered to the front door straight from our small local farm. It's different now. Much of today's milk (dairy) is simply not what it used to be on so many levels. And the recent issues with milk arise at every step from the farm to the market.

Start with the cows... we know that healthy foods come from healthy plants and animals raised naturally in their normal environment. Well, with "Big Dairy" that's pretty much out the window. Then during processing, pasteurization (necessary in Big Dairy" production) and homogenization destroy much of the health benefits of dairy. While we're left with a drink that is devoid of harmful pathogens, and no longer has the cream on top (a benefit for someone, I guess), it is now "dead" compared to it's raw origin.

The bad side of processing:

- Destroys beneficial bacteria and enzymes (aid digestion of milk)
- Destroys many vitamins and minerals
- Distorts the fats making them less healthy
- Causes xanthine oxidase release, a superoxide capable of much damage
- Proteins are denatured causing them to lose much of their health benefits
- Hyper-immunization, hormone use and the like with cows produce a milk with controversial ingredients in the final product
- Enrichment of milk often uses poor forms of nutrients that do little good for your health and can be harmful.
- And, by now you know, we don't advocate the use of any low-fat or fat free products and that includes milk.

After processing your left with only a distant and distorted representation of milk's raw origin. Honestly, this seems like

I'm one-sided in the end but I'm not. [In our house we do drink raw milk from a local farmer, and friend.] But, I think you do need to take an honest look at these issues when you consider milk. For my client's sake, initially, I am less concerned with dairy than I am with what is sold as dairy. Then, it's on to how you respond to it.

Clinically, many adults don't do well drinking milk, particularly the store-bought, processed, nonfat, white sugar water available to us. However, many people can tolerate and in fact thrive on dairy, especially cultured products like kefir, lassi, plain yogurt and cheese. Ideally these should be from raw milk or at the very least non-homogenized (also called Creamline) sources.

Your UP:

Whether you look good with a milk mustache depends on you.

1. If you drink milk, see if you can find raw dairy at a store or from a local farmer and give it a try.

2. Try different forms of cultured dairy to see if you handle them differently.

Section 7 Recap

1. We see how critical it is to stay hydrated and the many ways we can up our hydration (and nutrient) intake with broths, veggie drinks and super smoothies.
2. We are committed to drinking clean water

Resources and handouts for Charge UP can be found at: http://healthecoaching.com/charge-up-program/charge-up-additional-resources/

Section 8: Super Food Shift

How Super Are Your Foods?
Superfoods: Definition - A category of nutrient dense, vitamin and mineral-rich foods found in nature.

Nutrient-Density Diet: As boring a name as it is, it's about as close as I can come to a nutrition plan that works for everyone. Sadly, our foods have lost much of their nutrient density today so we need to proactively add diverse nutrients back... at every meal. Tremendous health can be gained by maxing out the nutrients in your diet.

Here are my top 5 Favorite SuperFoods:

- Homemade Vegetable and Bone Stocks - provide a large spectrum of vitamins and minerals - easy to digest.

    Great as bases for soups, grains, or as a warm drink.

- Coconut Oil - medium chain triglycerides which are crucial for healthy metabolism and brain function

    Cook with coconut oil, add to your smoothie.

- Dark Chocolate - Yes, Chocolate! The darker the better. We're talking at least 70% or better. Skip milk chocolate. Adds tremendous antioxidants to your diet.

Cocoa nibs have no sugar and are a little on the bitter side, but they add a nice crunch to your smoothies. Add dark cocoa to coffee. Enjoy small squares of dark chocolate regularly

- Chia Seeds - great for digestive health, high in protein, and healthy fats - using these daily will help insure you are detoxing.

    Add to your smoothie or make chia pudding

- Green Tea - full of antioxidants called catechins-- helps to regulate metabolism, boost immune system, prevent cancer. High in theanine for calming action.

    1 teabag, good quality - used throughout the day will increase antioxidants with each cup.

Your UP:

Max out the nutrients in every meal.

1. Choose a couple of these SuperFoods and begin to incorporate them into your routine this week.

How To Super-fy Your Current Diet

If you are eating from the Founder's Food* list, then most of your foods are already super. However, there are ways to max out the nutrients in your other everyday foods... only a couple simple tweaks.

The Nutrient Density Plan is too boring a name for a diet but it might be the simplest and most healthful perspective on nutrition I can endorse for everyone. It's simple, it works, and your body will thank you.

Despite the simplicity of the nutrient-density concept, don't be fooled – nutrition is complex, a realm for experts, really. Here's the good news, a "clean" body with an efficient metabolism is absolutely an expert in this area and, if given the right nutrients, will make most of the decisions for your health that need to be made. Most of us simply aren't giving our body the chance to show off its skills.

I was inspired to highlight a few ideas from the book, Eating on the Wild Side,* by Jo Robinson. She is also creator of the website, EatWild.com* – one of our most widely recommended resources for finding grass-fed, local and organic foods and farmers.

I compiled a short list – inspired by the book and straight from my personal recommendations to clients over the years. I love this stuff. Oh, and so will you… "nutrient dense" offers more robust, better tasting flavors that your body will love and thrive on.

Nutrient Density: **Simple ways to max out your diet!**
- Lettuce: The darker, the better (think red leaf lettuce) and you want to choose lettuce that has loose leaves, not coiled around each other like iceberg. Lettuce that is open to the sun will have a higher nutrient content. When you buy lettuce, as soon as you get home, wash it and rip it into pieces. The lettuce will start making more phytonutrients as a way to protect itself from the damage
- Apples: When choosing apples, choose the ones which are uniformly red or pink. The color is a

response to the sun exposure and the fruit will increase its nutrients

- Onions: The stronger tasting onions, the more potent antioxidants and immune enhancing properties they contain (i.e. Sweet Vidalia is lower on the list).
- Farmer's Markets: Farmer's markets and local farms are known for using different varieties of vegetables and fruits – so shop there, and when you see something unusual, buy it. Your body will enjoy the different spectrum of phytonutrients. It's also a great way to buy fresh, and seasonal products which will be more nutrient dense, taste better.
- Potatoes: potatoes if you soak potatoes before you cook them, it will reduce the starches and lower their glycemic load. The same goes for chilling the potatoes after you cook them. Dark, thick skinned potatoes are more nutrient dense.
- Tomatoes: The smaller and the redder the tomato- the more nutrient dense (think cherry tom). Cooking tomatoes longer than 30 minutes doubles their lycopene content.
- Carrots: Carrots are better for you when cooked in oil because it makes their beta-carotene (fat-soluble vitamin) more available to you.
- Veggies: To get the most minerals out of all of your veggies – add an acidic medium like vinegar or citrus.
- Blueberries: Cooked blueberries deliver more antioxidants than fresh.
- Green Tea: Using the same green tea bag during the day- each new cup (fresh water and same tea bag) increases the catechin (antioxidant) content.
- Variety: Variety is key to optimal nutrition – different colors, different varieties, always using new foods.
- Color: Deep rich colors, usually mean higher-nutrient quality. Every color offers a different

nutrient profile, so eat a rainbow (Not talking candy, here!).

- Priority: "Eat Me First" foods include artichokes, asparagus, broccoli, kale, leeks, lettuce, and spinach – nutrient density deteriorates quickly.
- Skins: Eat the skins of fruits and vegetables – packed full of nutrients.
- Shelf life: The longer the plant has been out of the ground, the more nutrients it has lost: Eat fresh and local.
- Purple Carrots: purple carrots are higher in anthocyanins – much better than typical orange carrots. When you see purple varieties, buy them!
- Grass-Fed Dairy/Meat: Grass-fed dairy and meats are high in CLA – a cancer fighting, fat burning essential fatty acid. Always look for grass fed milk, cheese, and beef.
- Eggs: Eggs should always be from pastured chickens, not vegetarian fed which is so popularly advertised. Chickens are not natural vegetarians. They need access to all kinds of food, including worms and insects so that they can have a wide range of nutrients. The slower and lower you heat an egg, the healthier it is for you – think hard boiled and soft boiled.
- Cooking Meats: Cooking meats longer and lower temperature also preserves nutrients and prevents some of the glycation products associated with high-heat/charred meats.
- Factory-farmed Meats: chickens, pigs, ducks, geese and cows are tightly packed into cages with no room to move, can't eat their natural diet, or even act like animals. The constant stress and poor diet create unhealthy animals who need medications. Besides animal cruelty, which is unacceptable, their meat and by-products lack

nutrients and essential fatty acids. Know where your meat is coming from!

To underscore the importance of increasing nutrient density any way you can I want to share a scaled-down glimpse of what we're up against. This is a broader issue that affects us all. If you ask a big tomato company what's most important in a good tomato. They'll say "weight" (They get paid by the pound.), then maybe "durability" (Has to make it to market in good shape), then "color" (People want it to look fresh). Lower down on the list is flavor and not even on the list will be nutrient density. I don't pass judgment as they're simply trying to run a solid business but I also can't ignore the impact on health. The ultimate "cost" in my opinion, besides mealy tomatoes is poor nutrient variety delivered to your body. Creating health, therefore, is similar to building a house with just a handful of nails, a few pieces of wood and a screwdriver.

So, I want you to take this list, use it.

These are just a handful of ideas and there are many more tricks you can try. So, expand the list.

Your UP:

Get more nutrient bang from your food buck.

1. Read the article above, get the specifics but take in the overall gist. Find your own ways to max out nutrients.

Super Spice-y

Clearly, not everyone enjoys spicy food, but there's tremendous health potential to gain from the seasonings in our foods.

The nutrient-dense profiles of spices have broad physical action but specifically I want to present their value as powerful antioxidants. In nutritional medicine there is a term called ORAC, a marker to measure and compare the antioxidant power of foods. To this day, with all of our fancy food technology and advances in food science, the foods with the highest ORAC remain in the spice cabinet.

Spices deliver powerful kitchen table medicine as antioxidants quench the damaging effects of free radicals (Short version: Free radicals cause damage to and aging of our tissues).

Here are a few of our favorites with high ORAC values.

- Turmeric
- Cinnamon
- Parsley
- Basil
- Ginger
- Mustard seeds

ORAC is not the only value of these herbs and spices as many of our natural anti-inflammatories and natural antibiotics contain blends of these potent medicines.

Other SuperFoods to incorporate:

- Unrefined Sea Salt*
- Apple Cider Vinegar*with "the mother". We like Bragg's
- Berry extracts high in anthocyanins like ProBerry*by Dr. D'Adamo and Dr. Mitchell's Fruit Anthocyanins by Natural Health
- Fermented Cod liver oil*
- Unfiltered, Raw Local Honey*
- Coconut oil and coconut butter*

- Grass-fed butter

SuperFoods are usually recognized as calorie-sparse but nutrient-dense.

Your UP:

Recognize the value of your spice rack. Spice up your health with flavorful seasonings... anytime, all the time.

1. This week expand your spice rack and try new seasonings.

- Add cinnamon and/or turmeric to your smoothies, or even your coffee.
- Use Italian seasoning - on everything, why not? Spice mixes are full of high ORAC spices.
- Slice ginger and add it to your teas, soups and juices for some kick.
- Maybe try making your own mustard from a mustard powder. Real mustard is much more flavorful (and spicy).
- Add unrefined Celtic (or Himalayan) Sea Salts. Over 80 micronutrients to fuel your CHARGE.
- Get wild and spice-y

I only offer that these SuperFoods are "unusual" in that many people avoid them for one reason or another. Perhaps you've never even heard of them, let alone tried them. Otherwise, they're not that unusual and they make great nutrient-dense additions to your diet.

In some ways these foods offer a spectrum of nutrients that we just don't get enough of from other foods and therefore can have huge impact on our health.

Unusual SuperFoods:

- Kombu - A mineral-rich sea vegetable that can easily be added to anything you're making - used in cooking, kombu delivers added minerals to your meal.
- Coconut butter or mana - Full of healthy fats, this "butter" is great by itself.
- Egg yolk - Yes, I said yolk... It's time to bring it back. Gone are the days we have to eat slimy egg white omelet's and forfeit the healthiest part of the egg... the yolk. This is where you will find the vitamins and the choline. Choline keeps cells strong and is a brain nutrient... I think we all need this!
- Fish roe - Rich in protein, amino acids and essential fatty acids and vitamin D... praised in other cultures as a perfect fertility food necessary for producing healthy babies.
- Liver (calf, chicken, cod) - Not everyone loves liver, but it is a superfood-- very high in absorbable vitamins-- including A, D and iron. It is a powerhouse. Liver should be eaten about 1 time per week and should always be from a clean, pasture-raised source. If you don't care for liver, you can get freeze dried capsules.

Make sure you know your source is clean, grass-fed and humanely raised.

Your UP:

Stretch your palate and your mind when it comes to foods... your body will thank you.

1. Pick an Unusual SuperFood that you might usually skip and add it to your diet this week.

- Roe: Select fish roe in glass jars. Eat it alone, on a whole grain cracker, with hard-boiled egg slices.
- Coconut Butter:* Ideal to stave off sugar cravings. Play with it on foods or eat it plain. Promotes satiety.
- Egg yolk: eat it with the whites, easy.
- Kombu:* add to grains, or soups while cooking.

Mediterranean Liver and Onions

Ingredients:

- 6-8 oz. liver
- 1 large sweet yellow onion
- 1 sweet red pepper
- Unsalted, Kerrygold (brand) butter (If you're local to South Carolina, find <u>Happy Cow Butter</u>)
- Worcestershire sauce or Balsamic vinegar
- Mushrooms
- Roasted garlic cloves
- Your favorite savory herbs.
- Unrefined Celtic Sea Salt

Instructions:

1. Cut 6-8 oz. of liver into finger-wide strips. Cut 1/2 of the sweet onion and 1/2 of the red pepper into strips.
2. Heat skillet at about 3/4 max setting on range – (or the max temp that you can cook at for 15 minutes without butter smoking).

3. Melt Kerrygold butter, 3-4 tablespoons (yes, that's a shallow lake). Add your favorite savory herbs and a pinch of sea salt.
4. Toss in liver, onions and pepper strips. Stir frequently, flipping strips over.
5. About 10 minutes into cooking, drizzle about 2 tablespoons of Worcestershire sauce (not much more or you'll get soup) over sizzling strips. Balsamic vinegar works too, if you add your own spices to taste. I like just garlic and oregano for liver.
6. Let go for another 5 minutes, flip / stir once or twice. Drop in mushrooms with a couple minutes left.
7. Done at ~15 minutes total, or when liver looks red-browned, not black (don't want shoe-leather).
8. Garnish (this is important) with roasted garlic cloves. You can also use some fresh or dried oregano. Season with additional sea salt if desired.

Adopted from: freetheanimal.com

Super Soakers

It's a simple, essential trick that you just need to know about. And, if you dig it, you can take it as far as you want to go. If you're like me, keep it simple and you're already doing great.

So nuts, seeds, grains and beans all contain anti-nutrients in their protective outer layers. These sinister-sounding nutrients (like phytic acid) protect these foods from various "predators" (like mold and insects) and provide antioxidant protection against degradation.

The issue for us is that when they're consumed, these anti-nutrients chelate (tightly bind) minerals, preventing their absorption. They also inhibit enzymes necessary for the digestion of dietary protein and carbohydrates.

Insert years of anti-nutrient consumption and you might find yourself with allergies, altered brain function, fatigue, hormone imbalance, digestive dysfunction or any number of chronic conditions as deficiencies compound and digestive stress accumulates.

Consider this: Research suggests for magnesium alone, we absorb about 60% less from our foods that contain anti-nutrients. If that doesn't do it for you, I'll just offer that magnesium deficiency is the most significant mineral deficiency in the US. And as a cofactor in almost every biochemical reaction in the body it means your body's not getting its job done without it.

So here's why soaking our nuts, seeds, grains and beans is so huge. It mimics the effect of germination:

- Neutralizes the anti-nutrients
- Activates and multiplies nutrients - increasing nutrient density
- Activates digestive enzymes in the food
- Improves digestion and nutrient absorption in the body

I told you I just like to keep it simple with soaking, but essentially, I add my grain (or nuts, etc) to a glass bowl, with filtered water (2 parts water to 1 part food) and soak covered, from the morning until time to prepare for dinner (or oftentimes, as little as 30 minutes while I'm prepping dinner). Those that are experts have wonderful guides with food-specific soak times (and sprouting times) and general setup, etc. so look around.

Of note: This time-honored tradition of soaking has been lost in big manufacturing so diets high in processed food sources of anti-nutrients like cereal, crackers, bread, nut butters, etc. can be very problematic.

Your UP:

Get soaked and feel the difference.

1. Experiment with soaking all your raw nuts, seeds, grains and beans. See if you can taste the subtle, fresh, "green" flavor of the activated food. Begin to make soaking a habit in the kitchen, not just an option.

2. Explore sprouting and consider giving it a try. A personal favorite is sprouted quinoa.

Not So Super Foods

So today, I thought I'd offer some of the most common "health foods" that tend to be not-so super for your health.

You can find better (hard to find) and worse (easy to find) variations of some these foods but we all just need to realize that, in general, they exploit one or another of our beliefs about healthy food without revealing what makes them a poor option for you.

Not-So SuperFoods:

- Sports drinks, electrolyte drinks, energy drinks - poor quality nutrients, high sugar, artificial sweeteners
- Trail Mix - we wish this was a health food-- most mixes are full of sugar, canola oil and processed salt

- Energy Bars - loaded with sugars and carbs, poorly absorbed nutrients and oxidized fats
- Frozen Yogurt - full of sugar (and often artificial sugar), chemicals
- Granola - high sugar, highly-processed and oxidized fats
- Instant Oatmeal - simply put, this is a sugar/carb bomb - last thing you should eat for breakfast
- Reduced-Fat Nut Butters - fat is replaced with extra sugars and carbs and any fat is left oxidized
- Veggie Burgers - highly-processed dead food, MSG, weird, non-food ingredients
- Egg white-only breakfast options - missing the benefits of yolk (vitamin A, D and choline)
- Egg and Butter Substitutes - these aren't actually foods
- Light/Reduced Fat Salad Dressing - high sugar (or artificial), highly-processed and oxidized fats
- Diet Drinks - low calorie at the expense of headaches, fatigue and weight gain associated with artificial sweeteners
- Fat-free/Reduced-fat Dairy Products - processing destroys any potential benefit of dairy
- Diet Frozen Dinners - the box it came in might be better for you
- Muffins/Bagels - high sugar, highly-processed and oxidized fats, not much better than a cupcake
- Orange Juice from Concentrate - don't be fooled, same sugar content as a soda
- Bottled Water - essentially unfiltered tap water, if in plastic then you get leached plastic chemicals

These are just a sampling but prove to be the most common culprits of the health food myth.

Food manufacturers love to play on our beliefs so it comes down to a little awareness and inquisitive approach to promises of health. A bit cynical but... real health foods don't tend to have as big a marketing budget as these Not-so Superfoods.

Your UP:

Don't believe everything you think about healthy food... don't get fooled by the promise of health.

1. Find actual healthy variations of these foods, if they exist, or skip them altogether.

Section 8 Recap

1. We learned about the super and not so super foods as well as ways to improve the nutrient quality of many foods we are already consuming.
2. We are incorporating super foods into our daily routine.

*Resources and handouts for Charge UP can be found at: http://healthecoaching.com/charge-up-program/charge-up-additional-resources/

Section 9: Stop and Go

Stop, then Go, then Stop

So it may seem strange to start off a module on exercise by saying, "Stop" (or rest), but that's exactly what we're saying.

As one of the more counter-intuitive insights about exercise, the value of rest has fallen victim to our "If a little is good, a lot must be better" approach to health. But, no more... we now know that proactively not-doing is perhaps the most important (definitely most overlooked) part of your exercise routine.

Those of you who don't care for exercise will love this well-researched and thoroughly-documented exercise phenomenon. But you might find the next sentence off-putting, so hang in there.

In fitness, the concept is referred to as rest-based interval training, high-intensity interval training (HIIT) or Tabata Training. This stuff always blows my mind because it works so well.

The idea is simple - you go hard and then you rest hard. Or... in the words of my colleagues and experts in this training "Go 'til you can't, rest 'til you can."

It is all about working hard, peaking your heart rate and then resting. And when we're talking working hard... a very effective workout can be done in as little as 4 minutes out of a 15-minute session at the gym (or your den, really). Sounds crazy, right? You see something happens with this kind of training that far exceeds the calorie burning potential of a day on the treadmill or stationary bike. For 10 hours after a good interval (Stop / Go) session, you continue to burn fat - loosely called "afterburn" (or Excess Post-exercise Oxygen Consumption - EPOC). Don't you love this!?!

You do not get this afterburn effect from moderate intensity long duration exercises like long distance running. So, no more hours on the treadmill or long distance pavement-pounding runs. Long gone are the Jazzercise days of the 80's. Now, we can just go hard, focus on rest and reap better benefits from our workouts in shorter time than ever. Nice!

Both aerobic exercise and weight training can be combined in this Stop / Go type of training. And, the simplicity of the approach allows for significant leeway - regardless of your conditioning, you can "go until you can't, and rest until you can".

Your UP:

Get a whole lot more (out of exercise) for a whole lot less (time).

1. Evaluate how Rest Based Training (RBT) can fit in your life... if you exercise, try it... if you don't, try it (of course, take any and all necessary considerations for adding exercise to your life, like asking your doctor).
2. Our colleagues at Metabolic Effect (www.MetabolicEffecct.com) have set the standard for RBT.

The Wanderer's Gift

I have always enjoyed exercise. In fact, I've probably needed it to function normally and feel a sense of sanity, particularly more in my younger years. Here's my biggest mistake: I never considered walking a real form of exercise... it was for de-conditioned, inactive or older populations. Was I ever wrong!

I completely missed out on the exceptional power of walking.

When we exercise we are in an elaborate biochemical dance - hormones and neurotransmitters in an intricate interplay. This hormonal "soup" dictates how well exercise works for us. Are we fat burning, muscle building machines or are we contributing to our stress load creating muscle wasting and latent fatigue?

One way to insure your Stop/Go (interval/rest-based/afterburn) training is working for you is to balance it out with walking.

Here's why.

- Walking relieves excess cortisol (your stress hormone).
- Walking, particularly outside, has been shown to lower stress, boost immune system and lower appetite.
- Walking balances out higher intensity exercise by minimizing the effects of cortisol (read: it increases lean muscle mass and fat burning).
- Appetite control- the conundrum with exercise in the weight loss community has always been that exercise increase appetite. Of course, wanting to eat everything you see is a challenge if you have fat loss goals. Combining high intensity interval training with walking is the best way to also modulate this appetite effect.
- Walking activates our primitive brain (from our hunter gatherer ancestors). Imagine how much we moved and roamed in those days. We get back to our roots, our primitive non-hurried, low-stress mind... so, walking

activates our parasympathetic nervous system (resting state)... instant meditation for the mind.

BTW - To be clear, when I am talking about walking, I'm not talking about fast-paced power walking. I'm talking about leisurely walking (wander walking) - makes sure it is at least 1/2 hour.

Your UP:

Incorporate the exceptional power of walking.

1. Start to incorporate leisurely walking into your exercise routine - at least 3 times per week for at least 1/2 hour.
2. If you are new to exercise and walking is your only form of exercise, alternate higher-paced walking days with leisurely walking days (and as you build up health and endurance, start incorporating higher-intensity exercise.

Go... Get To It.

What I think is hard to convey is that elite athletes and professional physique models are using this very approach to peak their strength, power, endurance and overall performance. You and me, we do it for health - balancing hormones, sharper mind, more energy, excess fat loss... you name it; it's probably better with a little exercise.

Today, I'm going to ask you to find 12 minutes to workout....16 minutes would be great but I'm not going to push my luck.

The intensity of these interval burst exercises increases as oxygen debt accumulates... in just 4 minutes. I want you to reach oxygen debt three times today and feel the difference.

The intensity of a routine is relative to our conditioning but we can all find a workout that takes our breath away in just a few minutes. Some of you may be shocked at how long 4 minutes will seem.

Another great thing... you don't need to head to the gym or change your clothes... do it anywhere.

Your UP:

Make time in your day to move... you only need 12 minutes.

1. Complete one 4 minute Tabata routine - three times today (At least an hour apart). You'll need a timer to track seconds.

   Routine: (complete 4 cycles in 4 minutes)

   20 seconds - alternating high knee raise*
   10 seconds - rest
   20 seconds - full body squats**
   10 seconds - rest
   Complete three 4-minute cycles today.***

2. Find 2 other days this week and put in the same 12 minutes. Find a new routine if you'd like (search "Tabata" or visit www.MetabolicEffect.com).

* like marching in place. opposite arm and leg in motion at same time. push yourself to get your heart rate up.

** clasp hands out in front of chest. legs shoulder width apart. bend knees, chest moves slightly forward as you drop your butt toward floor. elbows on inside of knees. When thighs are parallel to floor, return to standing, repeat. push yourself to get heart rate up. (If you have a history of back problems, hernia or other condition that may warrant caution, replace full body squats with jumping jacks.)

*** If you're a routine exerciser, define your own routine or search for one online that will offer a very short (4-minute), very intense workout leaving you in oxygen debt, begging for oxygen (and consider adding additional cycles throughout the day).

Get your Move on!

Stop... Until Tomorrow

Let me ask you something, "Do you wake refreshed, energized and ready to face the day?"

As you probably know, we simply don't get enough sleep anymore... in quantity or quality. We routinely squeeze extra hours from either end of our sleep just so we can fit our busy lives into each day. And, for the hours that we do sleep our metabolism, our minds, even our bodies are fitful.

But here's the thing: Folks who get adequate quality sleep live longer, have better memory, have decreased cancer and cardiovascular disease, are happier and are leaner than the rest of us.

So... back to our question. Your answer to it is the easiest way to assess whether you need to fix your sleep. I don't want you to miss the gravity of the question and your answer... so, don't think "need to" reads as "should".

Interestingly, the number of hours is actually less important than the timing of sleep. Melatonin production starts about 3 hours after the sun goes down. This is the best time to go to sleep. The anti-cancer, antioxidant, fat burning effects of melatonin happen 3 hours after the sun goes to bed.

I am guilty of this, but evening exposure to artificial light (from your screens, lamps, street lights, alarm clock, etc.) sends a signal to the brain to slow down melatonin production and puts the breaks on initiating sleep. Your brain doesn't believe it's night time and you've interrupted the vital cycling of this powerful hormone.

Hard to believe but perhaps the single best thing most people can do for their overall health is limit exposure to light in the evening.

Take Back the Night: Hormones and Your Sleep

Rest, a Lost Virtue.

Our modern, driven society downplays the importance of sleep. Busy has become a badge of worth but not without its costs. Indulgences aside we as a culture have more of a pass-out and come-to approach to sleep. While we love a good night sleep, we routinely squeeze either end of it for extra time, every day. But, what if a good night sleep was the missing link to your health?

Here is the typical scenario: after a busy day at the office, you race home, get dinner on the table, then maybe get the kids into bed. Now, your belly is full and the house is quiet. You may start to feel sleepy, but you push through a few yawns and get your second wind. Instead of honoring this quiet time and preparing for sounds sleep, we:

Get on the computer, catch up on missed work or maybe get social on Facebook and such.

Get on our phone and trance with some games or texting.

Throw on the tube for mindless TV zone-out.

All of these activities, relaxing as they are, change the daily rhythm of your sleep cycles.

Sleep, it Does a Body Good.

Our genetic physiology wants (needs) us to go to bed when the sun sets and rise when the sun comes up. Sleep is to be sound and restorative. Mornings are a time of inspiration and vitality where we jump up and have excitement for the day because our hormonal cascade from the evening before is right where it needs to be. How many of us go to bed when the sun sets and wake when the sun rises? When was the last time you jumped out of bed, energized and vibrant? How many of us get the type of restorative sleep that is necessary for repair, regrowth and healthy hormone production? (Quick gauge... how unreasonable did most of this paragraph sound to you?)

Melatonin, an Endangered Hormone.
It's during the 3 hours before midnight when the body naturally releases melatonin. Melatonin, a hormone produced from the pineal gland, is responsible for regulating sleep patterns. It's also a powerful antioxidant and helps regulate female hormone cycles.

So here's the problem with our nightly wind-down routine. The number one inhibitor of melatonin production is, perhaps you guessed it, exposure to light. Even the light from an alarm clock is enough to disrupt melatonin, so if you're stretching the day with full lights on staring at a screen, you're asking for a rough night sleep.

141

So here's why we like our screens at night. Besides perhaps tackling extra work, one of the reasons we turn on our screens is that the rapid movement of light releases dopamine in the brain. Dopamine makes us feel good and drops our shoulders a bit, but it's also very stimulating. Unknowingly (until now), we are stimulating ourselves into a fitful, rest-less sleep. Here's how powerful even the most minimal amount of light can be. If a client tells me they know what times they wake at night, I know that they have a greater sleep deficit and greater negative effects. The process of seeing just the light of the alarm clock in the middle of the night disrupts the vital but delicate melatonin pattern. These people have greater trouble getting a restful night and the negative health effects compound. If you must get up at night, stay in the dark (a helmet may be in order so you don't hurt yourself), and try not to stimulate your brain.

So here's the simple version. Your body is trying to release a hormone that regulates sleep cycles, repairs and restores cells after their daily grind and regulates sex hormone production but we are actively and directly blocking its action with evening exposure to light.

Melatonin is so crucial to health that when the body is not able to release melatonin at the appropriate time, the next attempt is earlier in the morning. Melatonin cycles back around in a desperate attempt to keep you healthy. When this happens early in the morning, guess what, you feel groggy! Yes, that foggy, slow, hit the alarm clock 10 times feeling is partly due to irregular melatonin production.

Melatonin and Cortisol.
Here is the other kicker, if you are not producing melatonin at the appropriate time, you are shifting toward cortisol production. Cortisol, your stress hormone, when over produced for too long does all kinds of "fun" things in the body. Let's take a look at a couple.

Cortisol and Weight / Excess Body Fat.
At the very least, excess cortisol cycling in your body boosts blood sugar as if you were eating jelly donuts all day long. You may be struggling with your weight and here's cortisol telling insulin to store everything you eat as fat (or even didn't eat in the case of the cortisol-driven "jelly donuts"). This is perhaps the ultimate failure of calorie-deficit, deprivation-type diets or simply skipping meals to lose weight. Cortisol, out of its love for you and desire to keep you alive, mobilizes sugar bombs all day and tells your body to store it all away as fat because for some reason food is not plentiful and you're likely going to need it later. Persistence of this complex and essential mechanism can ultimately lead to Type II Diabetes, metabolic syndrome and the like.

Cortisol and Anxiety or Depression.
Cortisol is part of the "fight or flight response" that keeps the body and mind on high alert in acute danger. When used appropriately, it's a beautiful mechanism designed to keep us alive. More commonly today, our persistently high cortisol lifestyles have us running from non-existent bears all day long. The result is constant tension, fear, negative thinking and ultimate exhaustion… a combo that further perpetuates the cortisol cycle.

Cortisol as Central to Female Hormone Balance.
PMS? Irregular cycles? Menopausal symptoms? Excess cortisol over long periods of time causes something called progesterone steal. Progesterone is one of our calming, fat burning, bone building, sleep inducing hormones. Because it balances out some of the harmful effects of excess estrogen, it is a key player in all kinds of hormonal regulation, even dysregulation. When the body is making too much cortisol, it starts to steal the precursors away from progesterone production. So that nice list of progesterone benefits is at risk when excess cortisol is cycling. Simply put, for most of us,

143

making enough progesterone is key to healthy hormones and quality of life.

Take Back the Night.
So here's the bottom line. When you're not sleeping well, you're just not you. Melatonin takes a hit and sets a cascade in motion that leaves us a mess. We need to re-evaluate our need for sleep...good quality, restorative sleep... and take back the night.

Where to Start.
Sleep hygiene is the first step.

1. Keep your bedroom dark and comfortable.
2. Don't use screens after the sun goes down.
3. Get sunlight during the day. You cannot mimic the powerful effects of natural light for sleep/wake cycles. You MUST get outside.
4. Go to bed and wake up at the same time, everyday, even weekends.
5. Proactively address stress. It can be as simple as a 30-60 minute wander walk.
6. Avoid sugar, alcohol and caffeine.
7. Diet rich in tryptophan.

Identify your food sensitivities and address them. This is perhaps one of the most overlooked aspects of getting good sleep.

Regulating your stress hormone, cortisol, is so essential that it almost goes without saying. Get to know your daily cortisol pattern based on how you feel during the day, Your Charge. What time of day do you have your best energy, when do you "crash", are you tired, yet feel wired, trouble falling or staying asleep? Look for your energy patterns during the day to get an idea of cortisol function.

Digging Deeper Cortisol:
Cortisol is the hormone we love and need, but when it's diurnal pattern changes, we can really feel the consequences in our daily sense of well-being and vitality. We think it is important to measure cortisol levels fairly often when you are struggling with a chronic health issue, optimizing your hormonal health for slowing the aging process, increasing fertility or wanting to function better in sports and recovery.

A 4-point salivary cortisol test* is the best test for assessing adrenal function. Standard blood cortisol levels are only accurate for severe adrenal medical issues like Addison's and Cushing's Disease. Ask your Naturopathic or Integrative Doctor about ordering this type of panel.

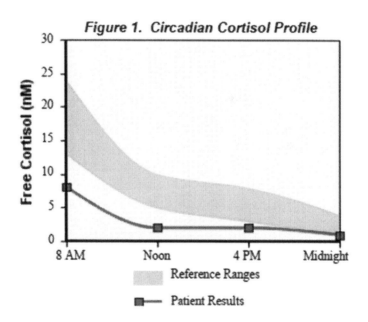

Figure 1. Circadian Cortisol Profile

This is a client with in a clear low cortisol, adrenal burnout phase. She is waking up exhausted, feeling run down and depressed most of her day and then not getting restorative sleep at night. Without adequate sleep, her adrenal glands cannot recover and she wakes the next day with low cortisol levels, feeling fatigued. She has also lost her zest for life, is steadily gaining weight, suffering from headaches and seasonal allergies. She has strong food cravings and an inability (and lack of desire) to exercise.

The goal of these simple recommendations is to help restore natural sleep cycles. But, life gets in the way of sleep hygiene and sometimes the negative effects of altered sleep cycles have taken their toll and more intervention is necessary via natural hormones and supplementation.

Clearly, we live in a modern society and while sleep hygiene sounds good, it is not always practical, but we must keep restorative sleep as a priority.

.

Your UP:

Get Sleep-y. Make quality restorative sleep a priority in your life.

1. For 7 days, commit to no screen time after 7pm.
2. Consider journaling your sleep pattern over this period.

(Believe it or not we don't really remember this stuff very well, so write it down.)

- How you fall asleep.
- How you sleep.
- How you wake.

3. Record any shifts in your Metabolic CHARGE.

Your Secret Fat Loss Formula

Stop: The secret fat loss formula

You probably know by now that we can't stand the nutrition and exercise dogma of "calories in, calories out". It's an over-simplified approach to weight loss that simply fails to hold water in a clinical setting. While it seems sensible at a glance, our biochemistry is much more complicated and far more dynamic than a simple math equation. So, "calories in, calories out" had a good run over the last 30 years but it continues to fail. Let's move on.

Whether we're burning fat, storing fat or maintaining is about hormones, an intricate dance of hormones. The result of the dance is dictated by the type of food we eat, how we break food down, the type of exercise we choose, and the amount of rest (sleep, relaxation, stress management) we get.

The right hormonal balance is at the core of fat burning. Sex hormones (progesterone, estrogen, testosterone), blood sugar hormones (insulin, glucagon), thyroid and adrenal hormones dance together each and every day and dictate what the body will do with fat.

So, the type of foods we eat (beyond just calories), how we Go and how we Stop orchestrate the hormone dance and will determine your secret fat loss formula.

Here's the most common scenario we see, why it fails and what needs to change:

I'd like to introduce you to Jill. Jill is a 55-year-old woman. She owns her own business. She is a caretaker and a go-getter in every aspect of her life. She comes in with a detailed food diary complete with portions and calories. She exercises 6 days a week alternating personal training with long distance running. She exercises long and keeps a strict low-fat, low calorie diet but her weight has stabilized shy of her weight loss goals. She carries most of her weight around her mid-section.

What Jill doesn't understand is that she has metabolic damage from years of her "high cortisol" lifestyle and exercise coupled with a low calorie, low-fat diet.

In order to reset her metabolism, Jill needs to back off on her workout, particularly her long runs. She needs more quality food with more quality fats, perhaps more calories, and she needs to rest more. Jill will find more fat burning benefits from choosing a yoga class over a high intensity session at the gym. She will shift into a fat burning state by adding leisurely walking and quality sleep to her routine.

Now that we know counting calories is not the way to lose weight or get healthy. Here's your new mantra for fat loss. "You get healthy to lose weight, not the other way around."

Your UP:

Count hormones, not calories.

If you have fat loss goals, start thinking about fat burning from a different perspective - a whole-body health perspective that focuses on the right hormone signals for fat loss.

What does your secret fat loss formula need? What's missing?

- More rest?

- Shorter exercise sessions?
- More quality food? (more fat, more calories, more nutrient-dense foods)
- Wander walking?
- Quality Sleep?
- Blood sugar control?
- Stress management?

Find Your Baseline

So today, we're going to go a bit beyond Stop/Go for those that have a good plan in place but they're still struggling to find the missing link in their fat loss pursuit.

Clearly, we believe there's more to a solid Stop/Go plan than just achieving fat loss, but similarly, there's a lot more to fat loss than just your Stop/Go routine.

Something that we incorporate in our Clean UP Program (formerly known as the 21 Day Metabolic Cleanse) is a daily physical modality. We have a host of different modalities to choose from, but the idea is simple - you have to move to get back to "baseline".

Baseline is loosely described as a place of stable, yet rhythmic, metabolic balance.

If you feel like your Stop/Go is solid and balanced, you're eating enough high quality, nutrient-dense foods but you're still struggling with fat loss, consider these underlying causes of fat loss resistance.

- Toxicity: Toxins are stored in fat cells. When the body is exposed to environmental toxins, it stores many of them away as a protective mechanism - gets them out of circulation. Wisely, the body resists breaking down these fat cells and their toxic cargo to prevent toxin release and their potential for damage to organs or other tissues.

- Food sensitivities: Eating foods that are not right for your body - results in a cascade of inflammation and water retention. Many "over fat" people are actually over inflamed/water retaining folks. This is an extremely common and likely cause for some excess weight.
- Hormones: There's a complex and intimate dance among our hormones. Adequate hormone balance, especially of estrogen, progesterone and testosterone, is crucial for fat burning. But, there are other players like ghrelin, leptin, insulin, cortisol, glucagon, growth hormone, thyroid hormones and more.
- Digestion: If you are not absorbing nutrients from the food you are eating a couple things happen. 1. Your body will drive cravings for more food in search of nourishment. 2. Your metabolism will slow as it's convinced it's in a relative starvation.

Restoring your baseline requires these issues aren't at play at the very least.

Digging Deeper: Your Baseline

Sometimes finding your baseline is simple. You need more rest and shorter exercise intervals. Detailed nutrition and hormone labs can give you some of the biochemical answers you need to overcome fat loss resistance into your ideal, healthful fat burning state. Full thyroid panels, adrenal testing, nutrients analysis and genetic panels can help you uncover your baseline.

Have You Maxed Out Your Energy Credit?
So people come to me all the time asking what they can do to get more energy. Here's what most of us need to understand about energy. Most of us have spent it all and have not done enough to fill the tank. It's easily likened to money in your bank account. You can't simply spend it. You have to earn it, too.

In recent years we've seen a surge in energy drinks and similar products that promise more energy, a clearer mind or sharper thinking. Sure they give you a quick boost but consider them like you would credit cards. When your bank account's drained, a credit card can cover you... you can just borrow what you don't have. But, we know the debt has to be paid down. It's the same with energy. If you borrow it, you have to pay it back.

When people are looking for more energy, they've usually tapped their energy account and maxed out their energy credit and they want the next boost. They're caught in a vicious cycle, their credit rating is junk and they're running out of options. The inconvenient truth is that by now the way to get the energy back is to pay down the debt and fill your energy account.

With the demands of life today I harbor no judgment. But reality... most of us are simply in some degrees of energy debt. The path to more energy is by earning it, paying down our debts and building our energy credit.

Outlined in previous weeks are steps to fill the account but the Stop in Stop/Go is about defining a program to decompress, unwind and rejuvenate.

Before we close out the week, I want you to be certain you have begun to incorporate a restorative routine to fill your account.

Your UP:

Earn energy, pay down your debt and build better credit.

1. Explore relaxing and restorative routines. Start with 10-15 minutes of "me time" each day... head towards 30 minutes a day, maybe an hour on the weekends. I might say that, if you don't think you have time or it's a waste of time, you probably need it most. We strongly believe in the power of mindfulness. When I try to sit quietly, my monkey mind freaks me out and I end up distraught, which is why I love the app, Headspace to guide me through my "quiet" time.

2. Get your Stop on:

- Journal in a notebook
- Epsom salt baths
- Massage
- Infrared Sauna
- Yoga
- Stretching
- Wander walking
- Breathing exercises
- Meditate
- Just sit and watch the day
- Find nature and hang out

Find what brings you a light heart and a clear mind and allows life to wash away for a period.

Digging Deeper: Sauna

An infrared sauna is not your typical coal burning sauna from the 1990's. While it does produce heat, an infrared sauna has the unique ability to penetrate through the skin into the muscle layer. It is this ability that makes hyperthermic conditioning a cornerstone of any detox program. We also consider it a cornerstone of overall health and longevity. In fact, when we first moved to the city and lived in a 500 square foot apartment, we promptly got rid of our dining room table to make space for our infrared sauna. This was over 8 years ago and we still use our sauna weekly.
Researched benefits include:

* increased insulin sensitivity (reduction in body fat)
* increased growth hormone (more lean muscle tissue)
* increased neurogenesis (growth of new brain cells)
* enhanced blood flow (stronger heart and blood vessels)

I could go on all day about my love for sauna therapy. We highly recommend High Tech Health infrared saunas. If you use my name (Dr. Sherri Jacobs) as the referring provider when you purchase, they will give you $500 off.
www.HighTechHealth.com*

Section 9 Recap

1. We learned Movement and rest in the right combination sets the foundation for fat loss, abundant energy and cellular repair.
2. We are incorporating rest based exercise into our life as well as time for us to recover, physically and emotionally.

Resources and handouts for Charge UP can be found at: http://healthecoaching.com/charge-up-program/charge-up-additional-resources/

Section 10: "Clean" Your Kitchen

By now, you should have a fairly clear idea of what you want to ditch in your kitchen, maybe it's already gone. Here's the thing... you can't always control the choices outside the home but you can and should make the right choices inside it. Your kitchen can save your life.

We apologize but we really couldn't ask you to take many of these steps at the start of the book... you would have wanted to know why, or simply glanced at the list and picked out what you wanted.

We've explored a lot since you started this book and hopefully you understand how we approach health and are willing to take these steps now.

It's time to approach the healing center of the home... the kitchen.

The overhaul begins: The DITCH in the KITCHen.

Ditch:

- All industrial cooking oils - vegetable, corn, soy and canola
- All processed foods with the industrial, processed oils: canola, corn and soy (as you already know, this is a tough one!)
- All low-fat and fat free products
- All butter substitutes
- All substitute meat products
- All obvious junk foods

- The trick foods which are junk foods in disguise: bagels, breakfast cereals, regular peanut butter, fruit juice and sweetened yogurt
- Sugar laden condiments like BBQ sauce, ketchup

This is just a brief recap, so take it as far as you need to go. Get these products out of your home and stop buying them. Remember, if it comes with a label, don't pick it because of the marketing. Go straight to the ingredients and test it against what you've learned in this program.

Your UP:

Take out the garbage in your kitchen - Ditch the foods that detract from your health and replace them with better choices.

All Cookware Is Not Created Equal

So the fridge and pantry are clean; whole, unprocessed foods are plentiful. Not that you won't ever have something processed, but they're no longer staples in your home.

So you have all of these wonderful, whole, fresh foods, but what are you using to cook them?

While it seems like non-stick cookware was the answer to every busy cook's prayers - less oil and less clean up - it turns out they're a terrible idea. Once again we got into a lab and created a shortcut but at the expense of our health.

PFOA, perfluorooctanoic acid, along with about 15 other types of chemical gases are emitted when cooking you cook with nonstick pans.

Peer-reviewed research suggests a link between these toxins and cancer, birth defects, flu-like symptoms, elevated cholesterol, abnormal thyroid hormone levels, liver inflammation and weakened immunity. Not to mention environmental bio-accumulation in the public water system and air quality.

If you're a bird owner, you likely know the non-stick issue well. The cumulative effect of these airborne toxins to the lungs of small birds is deadly. Big industry tells us, the use of non-stick pans is safe because we can handle a larger toxic burden load than a bird... so, cook on.

This doesn't sit well with us. Look at your children and other pets in the house - they seem rather small and delicate - yes? In my mind it shouldn't have to kill us to warrant a warning, killing small animals is enough for me.

The other cookware we have to ditch is aluminum pots, pans and utensils. Safety studies are contradictory but I don't think we should wait for them to agree.

What is certain is that aluminum leaches into our meals and excessive levels of aluminum are associated with Alzheimer's disease, kidney disease, headaches and osteoporosis. While there are multiple places of aluminum exposure in the environment we can't control, we need to limit our exposure in the kitchen.

Your UP:

1. Ditch the Non-stick. The good news is that we have broken the fat myth so don't be afraid to use traditional, healthy oils to cook with--no need for these non-stick pans!

157

2. Ditch the aluminum pots and pans

3. Ditch (or use sparingly) aluminum foil - definitely don't cook or wrap hot food in it.

4. Avoid processed foods (you're doing this anyway).

5. Avoid sodium aluminum phosphates. They are added to cake mixes, frozen dough, pancake mixes, self-rising flours, processed cheese and cheese foods and beer (in aluminum cans).

6. Avoid (or use sparingly) canned foods and drinks as the can lining leaches. (i.e. buy your beer in glass bottles)

7. Be aware: Some meds like buffered aspirin and antacids contain aluminum. As well, so do most toothpastes and deodorants (BTW-- deodorant has any ease transport system into the body-- the pores under the arm deliver right into the blood and lymphatic system).

Cookware We Love

Now, you know what cookware you shouldn't use... how about what you should?

We choose pots, pans, dishes, glasses, etc. for their stability, inertness, and (non-reactivity). Even my kids' drinking straws are stainless steel.

So... here are our favorites:

- Cast iron
- Ceramic

- Glass
- Stainless steel
- Enamel (Must be high quality and not scratched or prone to scratching. Caution: Do a little research as many do contain toxic metals like lead, cadmium, etc... of course these brands are not welcome in your new kitchen.)
- We use stainless steel spatulas, spoons, tongs and wooden spoons when cooking

We even use mason jars to drink out of - yes, we even use them as wine glasses... aren't we fancy.

Your UP:

There has to be a holiday coming so start looking for some new cookware.

Plastic Nation

You can tell from the title of this email but... we are a nation of plastics. While they have afforded us major conveniences and advances in industries like health care, they come at the expensive of health.

We went over this briefly before, but now we're going a little deeper.

Take a minute to think about your day and how often you come across plastics. Almost every food we buy comes wrapped in plastic, and before that food makes it to the store, it was likely processed in and through a lot of plastic. Cans and boxes are lined with plastics. Even the butcher paper for your fresh fish is lined with plastic. It's nearly impossible to avoid it for just shy of everyone. It's everywhere and with all of its uses, some might ask, "why would you want to avoid it?"

The greatest problem with plastics is that they leach gnarly chemicals into your food and drink. No doubt you've heard about BPA (Bisphenol-A), and perhaps, phthalates, the two most researched and recognized chemicals from plastic in our foods. These two classes of chemicals are known as endocrine disruptors or xeno-estrogens (And we feel that they're not alone. Regrettably, it is likely that BPA-free and phthalate-free products contain other chemicals we will soon know to avoid - at the moment the research is simply lacking.)

But simply put, these plastic chemicals interfere with our entire hormone system. This is not okay. Your hormones are essentially very powerful and rhythmic regulators of every metabolic action in your body - daily, weekly, monthly, yearly... across your entire life.

While it's near impossible to live a life free of plastics, you can and should take any steps to manage your exposure.

Here's the easiest... stop buying plastic bottled water, please! I see folks at the gym all the time who clearly care about their health, but 9 out of 10 of them carry a plastic water bottle (sometimes single use bottles, others are cheap reusable plastic). Why work against your workout (and ideals for health) by sipping on an endocrine disruptor?

(While beyond the scope of the program, there's also the significant environmental impact of plastic water bottles. Watch the movie Tapped, if you need a little inspiration to quit.)

Your UP:

Actively pursue plastic-free-ish living.

Visit www.EWG.org,* one of the best resources we know for clean living

Besides plastic water bottles here are some other great starts for plastic-free-ish living.

- Go for BPA-free cans* with any canned products.
- Do not heat anything or put any hot foods in plastic - opt for glass or ceramic.
- NEVER use plastic baby bottles.
- Use a silicone or stainless steel ice tray.
- Don't cook with plastic spatulas and utensils.
- If you use straws, opt for reusable glass or stainless steel straws.
- Don't eat microwaved popcorn and avoid fast food restaurants - wrappers and linings are plastic.
- We'll tackle microwaves soon but when reheating food in a microwave, cover with a paper towel, not plastic wrap.

Best Place To Keep Cookbooks

... is in your microwave.

Maybe you guessed but we're not huge fans of microwaves. I'm not sure I'm going to convince you to get rid of it, but we did several years ago and I think it was one of the best choices we ever made for our family's health.

The usual conflicts with microwaves regarding safety, health risks, or even benefits revolve around potential radiation exposure, changes in nutrient quality, carcinogen production and perhaps others.

I'm not going to lean on tons of research because it's full of conflicting findings. So, maybe it's personal bias but here's another time I won't for "industry" or legislation to decide for me. In the meantime, whichever way the research falls, I feel comfortable I've lost nothing for skipping the microwave and possibly preserved and gained a lot.

Here's why. Beyond the usual concerns, here's the reason I feel ditching our microwave was huge... to me, it's just not cooking.

There is something wonderful about preparing and cooking a beautiful meal. Maybe it's mental or subconscious or even "spiritual" but it seems lost in microwaving. Maybe it's a romantic notion but I feel that finding nourishment in a meal is more than taking an inconvenient break in my busy day to fuel up with the spectrum of vitamins, minerals and macronutrients. As we know (we explored this early in the program), our mindset and our circumstance greatly affect how our body responds to our food and how well the food nourishes us.

I feel that (if I'm given some leeway) I can translate the approach to microwaved nourishment into far greater generalizations for the way we're approaching our health and perhaps even our lives. Okay, bring me back.

I guess, just think on it.

Before I go, here's what I do feel strongly about regarding microwaves:

- Although microwave safe dishes are safe for your microwave, it doesn't mean they're safe for your body. Careful that they're not leaching chemicals into your food.

- Never microwave in plastic or covered in plastic.
- Most microwavable foods are too processed to have a place in your "new" kitchen.
- They make great bread boxes or storage for cookbooks.

Your UP:

Simply reflect on whether a microwave should have a place in your home and if it does, make thoughtful choices when and how you use it.

What's Lurking Under Your Sink?

Green is the new black, right? While being green was once for hippies, now it's gone mainstream. You can find green products almost everywhere these days.

If your cleaning supplies are not green, consider switching to more environmentally safe and health conscious products.

Our favorite clean living resource, Environmental Working Group (www.EWG.org), has a great guide to cleaners.*

If you're like so many of us, you may have a few green products to clean with but then there's that hard-hitting chemical cleaner for those really tough jobs! I get it. It's not my place to judge but we need to recognize that these toxic chemicals leach into the air we are breathing... through the container. It doesn't matter if their caps are sealed.

I say, if you're going to use them, get any harsh cleaners out from under your kitchen sink and put them away from the family's living space. Store them in a garage, a shed, in a container outside, even a basement or laundry room. You can get them when needed, but you're significantly decreasing your and your family's exposure to the off-gassing chemicals.

Consider this: these volatile chemicals (they're able to drift in the air like smells) have the ability to get to the deepest and smallest spaces in your lungs. This makes them especially concerning air pollutants and they are often readily absorbed into your body.

We love cleaning with watered-down distilled white vinegar and, to cut the smell and add to the cleaning properties, we add essential oils like lemon, orange, grapefruit or lavender!

Your UP:

"Clean" under your sink. Green your cleaners.

Kitchen Doodads I Can't Live Without
So, I love my kitchen. I guess you might imagine that but I really love it. But it's not the flooring or any fancy appliances; it's the culinary healing that happens there.

I believe deeply in the power of food, so I couldn't live without a good set of "tools". You'll find most of them are staples in any kitchen but in step with this week, they're specific for one or more qualities that support my healthy and healing kitchen. And anything that makes healthy living more convenient is a plus...

- Cast iron pans - all different sizes and shapes
- Glass baking dishes
- Mason jars for drinks, canning, dry storage, leftovers and soaking grains (all shapes/sizes)

- Stainless steel re-usable straws
- Bobble bottle brush for cleaning glass water drinking bottles
- Silicone ice tray
- Glass Tupperware-like storage containers
- Wooden Spoons
- Stone Mortar and Pestle
- Vitamix - powerful blender for shakes and soups
- Crockpot - always making homemade stock - no hassle
- Glass or stainless steel water bottles - I carry water with me everywhere
- Aquasana Water Filter* (or other) for drinking water, cooking water, and ice cubes
- Bamboo cutting boards
- Different sized cloth and fabric as napkins or for wrapping sandwiches, etc
- Cloth Tea Towels for cleaning up messes
- White vinegar, baking soda and essential oils for cleaning
- Stainless steel cooking tongs
- Glass pitcher
- Cordless stainless steel electric water kettle
- Stainless steel steamer basket
- Stainless steel colander and mesh colander
- Julienne peeler
- Stainless steel measuring spoons
- Glass measuring cups
- A great knife for each cutting need - good sharp knives will change your "cooking" life
- 20 qt. stainless steel soup pot
- Glass citrus reamer
- Salad chopper (looks like a double pizza wheel)
- Glass Pepper, Salt and Herb Mills

Your UP:

Fall in love with your new kitchen.

Section 10 Recap

Enjoy going through your kitchen and deciding what no longer fits into your healthy lifestyle. Simplify your pots, pans and cleaners. You do not need much, but you do need clean quality.

*Resources and handouts for Charge UP can be found at:
http://healthecoaching.com/charge-up-program/charge-up-additional-resources/

Section 11: Stress-Less

While this is the bonus section, it is actually the most important section of the entire book!

So, like many of you, I have an intimate relationship with stress. I enjoy the adrenaline of a tight deadline, a big presentation, challenging clients or interpreting difficult lab results. Each day and on weekends, I am a mother, a wife, a doctor, a business owner, and a persistent go-getter. I rely on a solid dose of stress hormones to keep me sharp and motivated.

However, when I go too hard for too long, riding the stress hormones without proper balance, stress turns into my worst enemy. The cortisol and adrenaline which I use and thrive off become too much. Then comes the neck tension, some nervousness, a racing mind and trouble sleeping. I know I've pushed my limit and stress has turned against me.

Similarly, my mom, one of the more impressive people I know, thrives off stress... until she doesn't.

I bring her up to demonstrate a point. When she crosses her stress threshold, she gets irritable, short tempered, and pushes herself harder, leaning into the stress. She goes into a "fight" mode, of sorts. I on the other hand go into "flight" mode. I recognize my tendency but I'd rather hide and retreat from the stress.

Perhaps we have adaptive responses having shared our lives together, but my point is that when we lose our balance with stress, we all have a unique response and unique presentation, or set of symptoms.

Another point to grasp is that a significant amount of stress comes from positive events. Easily one of the most stressful times in my life (causing significant stress-related symptoms) was around 2003. I had recently moved across the country to Seattle, had started medical school, had fallen in love and got married, purchased our first house, and we were having our first child... all within a couple years. All of the stressors were wonderful and positive (called eustress), but nonetheless, the highs (just like the lows) required cortisol and adrenaline and over time, I crashed.

So, now that you know about me (and my mom), this week we're going to look at you and how stress fits in your life.

Your UP:

Get to know your unique stress response.

1. Take an honest inventory of the stressors in your life. Write them down... the good and the bad.
2. Reflect on your stress personality. Are you a "fighter" or a "flighter"? Adrenaline Junkie? Workaholic?
3. Consider where your stress balance is and what it looks like when you've gone too far.
4. Check out one of my lectures on stress like Bear in Your Cave? ... Then Sip Tea,* when you have some down time.

Your Brain's Off Switch

Recently we were at a TEDx event and one of the speakers, Sundar Balasubraman said it perfectly, "our minds are like monkeys, but not just any monkey, a drunk monkey, a drunk monkey stung by bees."

Do you wish your brain came with an "off" switch?

… so after a long day you could simply hit the switch; the thoughts would stop; your shoulders would drop and you could just be. Sounds so peaceful.

"Remember you are a human being, not a human doing." ~ spiritual advisors since forever (I can't find original attribution).

Today I'm going to share what I do to flip the switch.

If you're like me, you often wish you had better control over your brain function. As a high achiever and highly sensitive type, I have a tendency to over analyze and over think. I'm deeply invested in the care I give others, in my clients' well-being and even what they think of me. This combination makes me well-suited for this kind of work; I'm very good at it. It's a joke to me when I have to turn in my continuing education hours annually because this is my life. I've said it before but I love what I do so much that I spend my downtime learning, analyzing and researching nutrition and naturopathic medicine – simply for the joy of it. I truly love it, but there's a risk. Flipping the "off" switch doesn't come natural to me so I could be headed for "burn out". Even the greatest strengths in excess can become weaknesses.

Bear with me (maybe you can relate) Most days before 6AM (when my husband finally opens his eyes), I have contemplated the purpose of my life while doing a little yoga, listened to a 60-minute podcast, poured over a few client plans, cleaned up my email, and packed lunches for the kids. It's a busy world in my head and keeping busy provides some relief! This is all well

169

and good. Professionally it's excellent, but the lack of balance is unsustainable.

Most people who know me would never imagine the pace at which thoughts race through my mind. I manage it quite well. I have to. As I said, I could be headed for burnout otherwise. Now let's see what we can do for you.

An overactive mind is the result of numerous issues, physical, emotional, spiritual, even cultural. Here are a few potential causes and potential remedies for you to consider. Keep in mind... you're unique; we need to respect that.

Why your mind races:

1. Gender: Some of us are "hardwired" to be caretakers (often considered a feminine skill) and this often extends well beyond the immediate family. As caretakers, we feel our place in the world and in the family unit is often about fulfilling the needs of others. There is no reasonable end to this task and over time our biochemistry may suffer. We become susceptible to burnout. Perhaps you've heard of the loosely defined Mama Bear Syndrome... a constellation of neurochemicals helps keep the female brain alert, active and ready for threats to the den. A hyper-vigilance and readiness to act presides. This worked well when there weren't so many mundane threats to consider like bank accounts, emails and recitals to attend.

2. Genetics: While the role of genetics is a very complex topic and our understanding develops daily, there are a myriad of enzymes that change the rate at which we

metabolize some of our precious neurotransmitters that affect thoughts, emotions, actions and reactions. If you are born into the world with a genetic tendency for some of the enzymes to work more quickly or to work more slowly, then you may find yourself more susceptible to varying levels of healthy brain chemicals. Gene variations coding for enzymes like COMT, MAO, MTHFR can change the way your brain behaves. The predisposition or propensity means you have to be more proactive about your physical and emotional health to balance the genetic tendencies toward an overactive mind.

3. Adrenal health: Your stress glands, called your adrenal glands, sit on top of the kidneys. They are responsible for producing cortisol during times of stress. Stress can be from emotions, poor food choices, environmental toxins, lack of exercise... the list goes on. Some of us are more susceptible to the ill effects of prolonged cortisol exposure and when the adrenals are not working optimally, symptoms like insomnia, anxiety/depression, fatigue, poor blood sugar control and hormone issues can develop. There are the environmental/external reasons which can tax your adrenals as well as genetic reasons that predispose you to stress overload.

4. Nutrients/Gut Health: B12, folate, B6, niacin, tryptophan, tyrosine, the list is a mile along. All of these vitamins and amino acids are necessary for balanced brain chemistry and they all come from the food you eat! And the food that you absorb! High protein, nutrient rich diets are imperative for a calm brain as is healthy digestion. The food choices you

make are as important as your ability to break them down. You must have good gut health to absorb nutrients from your food. And sometimes, that may not be enough, back to genetics, some nutrients are needed in high supply and you may not be able to get them in the quantities you need solely from the foods you eat. For example, with the genetic-based, nutrition related disorder, pyroluria, the body can become deficient in zinc and B6 and will undoubtedly cause an anxious mind as it depletes cofactors essential to neurotransmitter production.

Find your "off" switch:
Meditation is an essential tool for accessing your mind's off switch, but when your mind is overly busy, meditation can seem like a cruel punishment. Sit with your spinning thoughts? No thank you! I opt for guided mediation where someone walks you through deep breathing and awareness and not complete silence. Headspace Meditation App and Meditation Oasis podcasts are favorite resources. Other people discuss Getting into the Flow as their secret to quelling a racing mind. We really like the book Flow* by Mihaly Csikszentmihalyi. Personally, we have tried various meditation techniques over the years. The style of meditation that has worked for both of us is Vedic meditation taught by Emily Fletcher. We highly recommend her online training course through ZivaMind*

1. Exercise, oh sweet exercise. Nothing boosts serotonin and degrades adrenaline more effectively like exercise. Most of the time, I could care less about the physical benefits of exercise, will I look better in my

jeans or shed unwanted pounds... who cares! My brain needs the exercise, literally... without it, well, it's not pretty. Busy minds must move their energy and busy their bodies if they want to even consider finding their "off" switch.

2. Diet: A diet rich in protein and healthy fats is your best bet for supplying healthy brain chemicals. Your neurotransmitters are produced from protein breakdown and your brain is made up of 25% fat. Your brain must have these two macronutrients! Fats have been vilified for 30 years and, I am certain the costs for mental health have been significant. Consuming adequate quality fats cannot be overstated.

3. Nutrients to consider, consult your healthcare practitioner for guidance and safety.

o Magnesium: Calming to the mind and the body. Magnesium is the most widely deficient mineral in our society. The magnesium l-threonate form of magnesium is able to cross the blood brain barrier to protect neuronal health, and neuroplasticity (adaptability) while also calming the busy brain

o Theanine: The amino acid found in green tea has been shown to promote some of the same brain waves we use during meditation.

o The B-vitamins: These all have their place in brain health to varying degrees. Folate and B12 are needed for many of the genetic variants of MTHFR. B6 and niacin are essential cofactors in a myriad of brain functions like the production of calming neurotransmitters, GABA and serotonin.

o Amino acids: There are a variety of different amino acids (building blocks for neurotransmitters) like tryptophan, 5-HTP and tyrosine which are necessary for healthy brain function. Getting an amino acid panel done is a great way to see which ones might be right for you.

o Adrenal support: I think most of us would do well on adrenal support b/c we are all faced with so much stress in our modern world. Vitamin C, B5 and adrenal adaptogens like Ashwagandha are great starting places. I often recommend <u>testing salivary cortisol levels</u>* to see what your body needs.

Talk to your Naturopathic Doctor, Integrative Doctor or Integrative nutritionist about testing options which can help you find the best tools to calm your busy mind. Amino acids panels, adrenal panels, neurotransmitter panels, there are a myriad of ways to look deeper and find what your body actually needs. For instance, how your diet affects your genes* is one of the hottest topics in nutrition field today.

Time to Catch a Hormone Thief?

The body is so smart. When I try to consider all that it does (billions of biochemical reactions per second, a dynamic and rhythmic flow to it all - day to day, year to year), my mind collapses.

Here's just one thing that amazes me... an example of your body's inherent wisdom.

Cortisol, your stress hormone, is a life saver. For all that we might harp on it, without it, you would not exist.

Among other things, cortisol...

- Regulates blood sugar levels, insuring the brain and heart muscle get the right amount of fuel necessary to function.
- Regulates sodium/potassium levels for every single cell in the body, maintaining a perfect and very narrow pH range (sounds boring but your biochemistry doesn't happen outside the range).
- Balances the immune system and controls metabolic function.

Cortisol is perhaps the most fundamentally essential hormone in your body. So crucial in fact, that when cortisol demand and production is running high for too long (read unbalanced stress), your body literally steals precursors from every other hormone pathway in favor of supporting cortisol pathways. The other hormones are rendered insignificant when "survival" is on the line.

To me, this is brilliant... the body appropriately shifting its priorities when necessary. Under long term high stress, the body enters survival mode. The body has little need for any other hormone function at this point. So hormone production for something like procreation... no time for that! (Think: low libido, irregular periods and/or PMS, infertility, lowered thyroid hormone production, middle weight gain). Your calming, fat burning, sex-enjoying hormone, progesterone, is literally being stolen by your stress.

Do you suffer from any of these symptoms?

- sugar cravings

- irregular cycles or PMS
- joint pain
- low libido
- acne
- depression
- brain fog
- weight gain

Men-- guess what-- these all apply to you as well (except for the irregular cycles).

- But add erectile dysfunction and gynecomastia (man boobs, speaking less than professionally)

These symptoms are related to low levels of progesterone causing an imbalance in the estrogen to progesterone levels.

And while we're focusing here on progesterone, every hormone in the body can be "stolen" by stress. Reasonably, deficiencies of other hormones would reflect in related symptoms.

The great news... if you stop the thief, every other hormone system will eventually rebound. Very nice! So think on this. If you have symptoms related to some "deficient" hormone, you may need to go after the stress to find any sustainable relief.

Your UP:

Play detective and stop the hormone thief.

1. Women, keep track of your monthly cycles AND your CHARGE. After a few months you might be surprised to see the correlations between your monthly cycles and energy, mood, cravings and sleep.

Digging Deeper: Hormones

Ever since the Nurse's Health Study when we found out some troublesome news about hormone replacement therapy, there has been a great deal of controversy over who should be on hormones and their level of safety. It appears Bio-Identical Hormone Replacement Therapy, the naturally derived hormones which mimic your own hormones, are safer. They are definitely necessary for some women to improve quality of life when going through menopause. We really like to look closely at hormones in relation to your CHARGE, but we don't always rush to use hormone therapy. There are many non-hormonal ways to balance hormones before having to give a hormone directly. We think it is important to test and not guess when it comes to hormone therapy. For women who are menstruating, we love taking a month long salivary collection called a Female Hormone Panel- FHP.* This is a beautiful way to see what is happening with estrogen and progesterone throughout the cycle instead of the conventional method of testing 1 single day in the cycle. As we women know, hormones (and symptoms) change from day to day during a cycle!

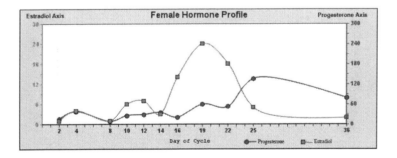

Month long female hormone panel (FHP): Once women get this panel done, we can combine it with their CHARGE to get a clear picture of hormone related symptoms.

Another favorite test for looking at all of the hormones in the body and how you are breaking them down is the <u>DUTCH test</u> (Dried Urine Testing for Comprehensive Hormones).* This test is perfect for pre-, peri- and post-menopausal females. This test accurately measures hormones as well as their metabolites. We can see how your sex hormones correspond to your stress hormones and how you are breaking down your hormones.

The Genetics of Stress
"Is it nature or is it nurture?" ... the age old question.

For us, regarding health and disease, it's clear there's almost always a mix of the two. However, with stress, there's a STRONG genetic component (i.e. nature) affecting how we cope and adapt.

While genetics was a dreadfully boring chapter of biology class for me, it has taken an exciting turn - very, very recently. I want to be very clear because this stuff is essentially "hot off the press" and flies in the face of older teachings on genetics. We now know that just because something is considered genetic (i.e. It's in your genes) does not mean it has to be your life's burden.

I want to share a personal story that helps convey why I love this new take on genetics.

So... it disappoints me when I look back but, early in my clinical rotations in naturopathic medical school (and with my BS in Psychology), if a client complained of anxiety or depression, I considered it simply a thinking problem, perhaps a world view problem or such. But, the budding practitioner in me got a slap in the face when I had my first bout with "paralyzing" anxiety.

When I experienced it for myself, the very physical nature of the experience, it became clear to me, my anxiety developed in the realms of my biochemistry, physiology, and neurochemistry. My feelings were being driven by something and my emotions and mental state were simply along for the ride, a reflection of the internal state of things.

I started looking into the genetics of anxiety and had my first clinical breakthrough when I started screening anxiety folks for a genetic condition called Pyroluria. Pyroluria is a nutritional disorder (which sadly often undermines its credibility) that can manifest as debilitating anxiety. Interestingly, and to the point of this email... this genetic condition need never rear its head if those with Pyroluria simply maintain adequate levels of a few specific vitamins and minerals. (If you're interested in Pyroluria, here's a deeper review I wrote for a clinical journal:

Whether pyroluria is an underlying cause of your anxiety or not, I hope the message is clear. Nutrition plays a significant role in your health and well-being.

Pyroluria: A Cause for Anxiety

A notable client comes through the door that has been anxious most of their lives or suffered frequently from episodes of nervous exhaustion. Their anxiety has become enveloping since a major life transition. Anti-depressants and anti-anxiety medications have not offered lasting relief. They are usually perfectionist and highly creative but carry around a significant degree of inner tension and fear. Since anxiety has become a common condition in our modern world, most clinicians find it a rarity when someone does not check the stress/anxiety box on their intake questionnaire. It is pervasive. As Naturopathic Physicians, we offer anxiety sufferers lasting relief by uncovering the underlying biochemical causes of the distress.

One biochemical cause of anxiety is a controversial and understudied condition which has significant implications in the treatment of anxiety; pyroluria. First discovered in the 1950's by Dr. Abram Hoffer, pyroluria is a genetic condition of altered hemoglobin breakdown resulting in a depletion of vitamin B 6. Without adequate B6, the body is not able to convert Tryptophan to serotonin. In the absence of adequate serotonin levels, many different psychiatric disorders, like anxiety, develop.

A normal by-product from the breakdown of hemoglobin, kryptopyrroles are found in elevated amounts in people with this genetic abnormality. As the pyroles are being excreted from the body, they bind two important nutrients; Vitamin B6 and Zinc. This relative deficiency results in a myriad of different symptoms that wax and wane over the years depending on someone's level of stress. Pyroluria is marked by symptoms of inner tension, nervous exhaustion and fearfulness.

Vitamin B6 is necessary for the conversion of tryptophan to the neurotransmitter, serotonin, protein and carbohydrate metabolism and a healthy immune system. Zinc regulates insulin activity, acts as a powerful antioxidant and regulates gene expression.

The combination of depleted B6 and zinc is a disaster for mental health. Both nutrients are essential for healthy brain function. Dr. Joan Larson, founder of Health Recovery center and author of Depression Free Naturally explains the role of B6 and Zinc in the following way. "B6 is the co-enzyme (meaning it is absolutely essential) in over FIFTY enzymatic brain reactions where amino groups are transformed or transferred. B6 has an important role in your nervous system's balance. It is required to utilize protein for energy. Brain depletion of dopamine and serotonin occur without B6, creating ongoing anxiety and depression. Zinc deficiency also results in multiple disorders. The brain uses at least sixty zinc enzymes so zinc deficiency has a marked effect on mood states. Anxiety and depression have been observed in clients who develop zinc deficiency from intravenous feedings. These clients experienced prompt relief from their acquired depression after zinc was supplied"1

Pyroluria Testing

Dr. Larson recommends the use of Bio-Center Lab as the only reliable lab for testing. The test is inexpensive and can be ordered directly by the client. The lab will assess the level of pyroles found in the urine. Results from 10-20mcg/dl of pyroles are considered borderline. Above 20mcg/dl is considered positive for pyroluria.

Because of the low-cost and ease of the test, I frequently recommend it when I am working with a client who complains of anxiety. A positive test insures compliance with the protocol.

181

Most "pyrolurics" have gone undiagnosed for many years. Due to the constant anxiety creating surges of cortisol and adrenaline, it is imperative for the clinician to also treat the adrenal glands. An adrenal stress index is warranted for a complete evaluation of a pyroluric client.

Pyroluria Screening
Pyroluria Screening Questionnaire: (sample)

1. Do you tend to skip breakfast or have morning nausea?
2. Do you tend to be anxious?
3. Do you have other members in your immediate or extended family with schizophrenia?
4. Are there members of your immediate or extended family who have committed suicide?
5. Do you have white spots on your nails?
6. Did you get a "stitch" in your side when you ran as a child?
7. Did you have moderate to severe acne as a teenager?
8. Do you have pain or creaking in your knees?
9. Do you have cold hands and feet?
10. Do you have stretch marks as an adolescent or adult even without a large weight gain or loss?
11. Are your teeth or were your teeth before orthodontic treatment crowded with teeth growing over teeth?
12. Did puberty start a little later for you than others?
13. Are you easily tired?
14. Do you tend toward apathy?
15. Do you have a tendency toward iron-deficiency anemia or test borderline?

16. Do you have eczema or psoriasis?
17. Do you have tingling sensations or even tremors in your arms or legs?
18. Do you tend to have paler skin than other family members?
19. Do you tend to get overwhelmed in stressful situations?
20. Do you have trouble remembering your dreams?
21. Are you now or have you been a vegetarian?
22. Are you now or have you before been an alcoholic?
23. Do you find yourself socially withdrawn and dependent fairly strongly on one person?
24. Poor short term memory?
25. Poor ability to cope with stress?
26. Mood swings or temper outbursts?
27. Much higher capability and alertness in the evening compared to mornings?
28. Sensitive to bright light?

Published in NDNR March 2010 by Dr. Sherri Jacobs

Now I'm several years into practice and we have much more information about the genetics of stress... as in, how your body handles it and what you, uniquely, can do to manage it. For example, the MTHFR (methyltetrahydrofolate reductase) mutation and related SNPs (Single Nucleotide Polymorphisms in gene sequencing like COMT, CBS and MaO) play a critical role in how your body produces and breaks down stress hormones and neurotransmitters. If stress is your thing, imagine what you could do with this type of information. That's the great thing. There's so much you can do!

Your UP:

Stress and YOUR stress response may be defined by the expression of your genes and you may be able to "rewrite" the definition.

1. Consider your family's "stress genes" and explore whether you need to break the cycle by positively influencing how your genes act.

2. There is a fascinating video on PBS* about the emerging view of genetics (That may sound boring... I get it but the implications for you and me, even future generations are mind blowing). We need to grasp that every aspect of our life experience (including diet) influences how our genes behave.

Baseline Bliss

So while we've harped on stress a bit this week, stress is a highly adaptive mechanism we should be thankful for. If we didn't have our intense stress response, we wouldn't have been around for very long as a species.

Let's go back a bit to see how it serves us. The hunter gatherer period lasted about 1.8 million years. We lived in societies which were fairly nomadic. Hunting and gathering food was of top priority for survival. We walked and moved around a lot, had relatively low daily stress and the stressors were rather limited. The general experience is what I refer to as "Baseline". We were constantly moving our bodies, we focused on food and we had relatively few outside worries. (I know it sounds simplistic but only by comparison with the complexity of our lives today.) Day to day, stress hormones were relatively low and consistent until a threatening bear came out of the woods.

On sighting the bear, the body enters a physiologically-driven survival mode, instantly - nerve signals stimulated by your senses notify the adrenals to release a surge of adrenaline and cortisol to prepare the body for fighting, fleeing or freezing (playing dead).

Instantaneously...

1. Eyes dilate.
2. Digestion stops. Metabolism alters to maximize blood sugar and blood oxygenation for energy production in the brain and skeletal muscle.
3. Heart rate increases to pump oxygenated blood more rapidly.
4. Blood pressure increases to better infuse tissues.
5. Air ways dilate and breathing increases to meet heightened needs for oxygen.
6. Nerve signaling heightens in the brain and muscles for fast thinking and quick action.

But as soon as the danger passed, the calming component of the nervous system kicked in and homeostasis was restored... life was good. That experience of "life is good" is "Baseline" - simple, peaceful, relaxed, no danger in sight.

Fast forward to today. While it's pretty rare for most of us to encounter a mad real bear during our day, we have significantly more persistent, often intangible, daily stressors that aren't too different. Essentially, today, we're running into bears all day, every day. You see, here's the great challenge with our incredibly evolved stress response. It really doesn't know that the Monday morning rush hour, next week's rent and a job interview are not bears. It receives the same stress signaling as if from the bear and sets off the cascading stress response in preparation for fight, flight or freeze.

But now where has our baseline gone? When during the day do most of us have that peaceful, relaxed, and quiet mind - stress-free without a care in the world except what to eat for lunch? How many times in a month or even a year do you feel like that?

The result... the overwhelming majority of us are living in the midst of a constant, low level stress response. We've adapted some to the persistent stress but we're rarely, if ever, reaching Baseline.

Here's the cost to our health (Not surprising in light of the list above):

1. Digestion is chronically slowed down. It persistently under-functions. (We know the costs from section 2.)
2. Blood circulation suffers.
3. Heart rate and blood pressure remain chronically elevated.
4. Over-breathing creates feelings of lightheadedness, anxiety, spacy-ness and muscle tension.
5. Blood sugar control seesaws as it peaks and drops and wreaks havoc on the body. (weight gain, insulin resistance, irritability, fatigue, insomnia, stress)

Baseline is essential to set us straight.

Baseline--what is yours? Walking, prayer, meditation, baths, massages. Everyone is unique in what gets them back to baseline. What brings you back.

For the next 7 days, you need to do whatever brings you back to baseline for 15 minutes EACH day. Does your CHARGE change at the end of the week?

Your UP:

Experience Baseline.

1. Identify what you need to get back to baseline and get to it. Everyone has their unique favorite. What's yours? If you don't know, start with wander walking (walk without an agenda) - it works for everyone. If it doesn't seem to work for you, you may actually need it more.

   - Walking
   - Prayer
   - Meditation
   - Baths
   - Massages
   - Reading for pleasure
   - Journaling
   - Whatever... find your own.
   - (TV, surfing the internet, etc... do not count... they're actually quite stimulating.)

2. For the next week, hit your Baseline for 15 minutes each day.

3. See if your CHARGE changes by the week's end.

My Favorite Stress Relievers

Like you, I have my fair share of stress. I like to think that I manage it okay but as I told you, I can tend to ride the stress too long. So, I have a few favorites for de-stressing depending on the situation.

One thing I find works well when I'm stressed is to get out of my mind and into my body. I like a book called <u>You Can Feel Good Again</u>,* by Richard Carlson with its simple yet powerful message - Change your thinking and you can change your life.

We've all heard this before (not to discount the message) but the book clarified a simple practice that I found worked really well for coping with stress or negativity. If I can just get out of my head for a bit, or simply, not dwell or overthink, the stress of the situation drops considerably. Perhaps the stressor hasn't changed by any stretch but the experience of my situation becomes so much more manageable.

The easiest way for me to get out of my head is to get into my body... become physical... "Do" instead of "think". Seems overly simple but it works.

So anyway here are a few specific, favorite stress relievers...

- Wander walking - out of my head, in my body, enjoying the moment
- Essential oils - diffused in the air. Works deeply but better for me as a preventative.
- Rescue remedy - liquid, under tongue for "intangible" stress. Good for acute stress.
- CES Treatment - Cranial Electrostimulation. Sounds creepy but it's not. Promotes relaxed alertness
- Lightbox - Full-spectrum sunlight lamp in morning. Elevates serotonin. Helps set daily hormones.
- Epsom salts -In a bath, deep muscle relaxation and detoxification. Soothing, quiet "me time".
- Yoga - Get into my body.

Nutraceuticals: Recommendations are based on lab testing demonstrating specific types of irregular adrenal function.

- Adrenal adaptogens like Ashwagandha and Rhodiola
- Licorice tea or licorice extract
- Vitamin C
- Hormone precursors like DHEA and Pregnenolone
- B vitamins (the right forms, of course), pantothenic acid is particularly important.
- Phosphatidylserine

Your UP:

"Lose Your Mind"

1. Perhaps try some of my favorites but figure out what it takes for you to get out of your head and into your body. And, see how it works for you. You may only need 5 minutes to decompress and if you find what works for you... you can always find 5 minutes.

Gratitude

So research suggests that expressing thanks may be the simplest way to feel better.

The Greater Good Science Center at University of California, Berkeley reports that people who practice gratitude consistently report a host of benefits:

- Stronger immune systems and lower blood pressure;
- Higher levels of positive emotions;
- More joy, optimism, and happiness;
- Acting with more generosity and compassion;
- Feeling less lonely and isolated.

At the very least gratitude is worthy of a good luck so I want to share a story I've always liked. It's fairly hypothetical but I think it conveys a great message we can work with.

So here goes:

Take 100 random people and ask them to take all of their problems, all their stresses and all the negativity in their lives and make a big pile out of them, on the floor for everyone to see. Then ask the people to walk around the piles and consider them. Have them go pick the pile of problems that they would like to have for their own. So the story goes that they would each go back and pick up their own pile. With the magnitude of everyone else's struggles in plain view, ours seem less daunting.

Why I like the story is because naturally, it's easier to be thankful for the good stuff in life (be sure that you are.). But, it's the "bad stuff" that impacts our health so negatively and the act of being thankful for them can do wonders for zapping their power over our lives and our health.

Interestingly, most of us seem to have a mild but innate discontent for where we are in life and what we have. This subtle nagging seems to be designed to keep us as individuals and a species moving forward, ever in pursuit of bigger and better things. On most days this serves us very well, but there are those days, even months or years, where we seem to be beaten down by it. I would offer that gratitude may be the most suitable start to get out from under it.

Your UP:

The fastest way to find everything you want out of life is to be thankful for what you already have. For at one time, it was all you dared hope for.

Practice gratitude today, and tomorrow... and then the next day...

This is a beautiful place to end our book...with gratitude.

Thank you for taking the time to Charge UP.

Made in the USA
Columbia, SC
19 July 2017